I0840243

PARASITES - YOU NEVER KNOW WHAT'S LURKING

30-Day Parasite Treatment Plan

DUROLLARI

Copyright © 2019 Durollari

All rights reserved.

ISBN: 9781710109429

DEDICATION

I dedicated this book to my grandmother Demire, my mother Nedime, along with my father Dr. Guri, and my lovely eternal princess Dbborra.

Consult Your Physician or Health Care Provider

Our intent is NOT to replace any care or relationship that exists or should exist between you or your clients' medical providers or mental health providers. Always speak with and seek the advice or your/their physician/doctor or other qualified health professionals regarding any questions or concerns about your/their specific health situation or concerns and before taking or changing any medication, nutritional, herbal or homeopathic supplement or other treatment and lifestyle habits. If you are under the care of any health professionals (or should be), we strongly encourage you to discuss modifications in your diet, lifestyle, exercise program, nutrition, stress management or use of other healing modalities, detoxes, supplements, vitamins diets, meditations, yoga, deep breathing or other aspects of a weight loss, healthy eating, exercise and/or lifestyle program with them prior to making any changes, and never discontinue or reduce prescription or other medications without consulting your doctor or pharmacist. If you or your clients have any health concerns or suspect that you have a medical problem, you should consult with a healthcare professional promptly. Do not disregard professional medical advice or delay in seeking medical advice or care because of something you have read or heard on this book or Products.

CONTENTS

ACKNOWLEDGMENTS

First, I would like to thank everyone for purchasing this book; also, I would like for everyone to understand the rationale and importance of publishing this book is solely to inform and help people infected with parasites. Like most people, very few know much about parasites, while there are very little public discussions concerning parasites. The media and the public health agencies provide very little information concerning the epidemic of parasites in our daily lives, it is like out of sight out of mind. It seems like no one is concerned enough to dig in and truly investigate and learn about parasites and their effects in our daily lives. It is also possible that in general, people do not want to think of the possibility that they may have parasites lurking inside their intestines and within their bodies.

Like most, people in general are afraid, and I certainly don't blame them, of the unknown and lack of Education and knowledge when it comes to parasites. Unless one has been clinically diagnosed and infected with parasites, it would have never crossed an individual's mind to study and or think about parasites. Therefore, I decided to write this book to inform the general public, while providing a road map with a logistical plan in treatment and eliminating parasites. When faced with the reality of being infected with parasites, it is imperative to take proper measures in eliminating parasites in the shortest amount of time possible. Without this knowledge, it can take years, and in some cases, individuals do not eliminate parasites from their body. This 30-day parasite treatment will provide a logical and systematic approach. Most fail because of a lack of knowledge and or willingness of will power and ability to research, study and experiment; the real power lies in the logical steps one takes to eliminate parasites. Being emotional and or afraid does nothing, and a more logical and systematic approach is the smarter choice of action in ridding of parasites.

Potential medications for treating parasites such as Blastocystis include antibiotics, such as Metronidazole (Flagyl) or Tinidazole (Tindamax). The physician additionally, prescribes the following combination of medications, such as Sulfamethoxazole, Trimethoprim, Bactrim, Septra, and including Antiprotozoal medications, Paromomycin, or Nitazoxanide (Alinia).

Treatment Plan List:

Prescription: Metronidazole (Flagyl) – 250 mg tablets each. Take 3 tablets by mouth three times daily, total 750 mg, for 30 days.

Essential Oils

Clove Essential Oil (Organic if Available) 4 ounces
Oregano Oil, Wild – 4 ounces

Olive Oil (Organic) 32 ounces

Green Tea
Black Tea
Black Coffee
Peppermint tea

Parasites Treatment Steps

Make a list of everything that is needed for the 30-day treatment of parasites, specifically blast sites.

Ensure you speak with your doctor concerning pharmaceutical protocol for parasites, and most doctors prefer a 10-day treatment antibiotic. My recommendation is to speak with an infectious disease physician concerning a more extended protocol of medications, and a better protocol would consist of a 30-day treatment plan of antibiotics, specifically Metronidazole, 250mg tablets three times a day. Treatment of parasites is a severe matter, and an individual infected with parasites should take this very seriously, at the same time do take a logical and scientific approach towards treatment and elimination of parasites.

The multi-dimensional approach is recommended towards treating and eliminating parasites, this plan consists of a pharmaceutical protocol prescribed by your doctor, several non-medical use of traditional herbs and essential oils, to include a restrictive diet, and fasting protocol during the entire 30-day program.

Step 1: Arrange an appointment with a primary care provider to accomplish a parasite stool test with a local lab, such as Quest. A fecal (stool) exam, also called an ova and parasite test (O&P)

Step 2: Once the lab reports are received, and the parasites are identified, your primary care provider will give you a referral to see an infectious disease specialist.

Step 3: With the consultation of your infectious disease doctor, work to create and inform your doctor that you would prefer a more extended pharmaceutical treatment plan that will consist of 30-days. Inform your doctor that a more aggressive approach towards treating in eliminating parasites should be more effective, rather than a 10-day antibiotic treatment plan. In the decision-making processes, considering the persistence of parasites and the difficulty of eliminating them it only makes sense to use a longer treatment plan.

Step 4: You will need to order approximately more specifically at least 1 oz of clove essential oil and 1 oz of wild oregano oil, but I recommend purchasing 4 oz of the clove oil and 4 oz of the regular oil in order to have plenty on hand for your treatments and elimination of parasites from your body.

Step 5: Eliminating parasites is not an easy task, and one must be psychologically and mentally prepared, while at the same time work in a logical way; think of it as you are going to war and be mentally tough for what lies ahead. Create a road map, outlined in a written journal that must be accomplished day-by-day for 30 days consistently and as accurate as possible. Make sure you follow this manuscript and do continue to conduct further research on your own, and scientifically annotating the findings in this manual.

Step 6: Keep in mind the approach that has been taken, and this manuscript concerns two types of parasites, which one is Blastocystis, and the other one is Adina parasites. There are hundreds or more of different parasites that exist, and more research will have to be conducted concerning each other parasites and what approach should be taken. Based on my experience, if the combination of the pharmaceuticals and essential oils, along with the proper diet and fasting periods, it only makes logical sense that this approach would work for many other parasites. Again, work closely with your medical provider and think of it as a team effort between you and your doctor. Therefore, it is essential to keep a written journal and in order record what works and what does not.

Step 7: Once the clove and oregano essential oil has arrived, purchase high quality 32 oz bottle of olive oil, using a dropper extract 1/2-ounce clove oil and 1/2 ounce of oregano essential oil and then place inside the olive oil bottle. Once the mixture is completed, shake the bottle well and store at room temperature.

Step 8: You will need the following foods for the next 30 days: onions, green onions, garlic, bitter greens, sauerkraut, pickles, sardines, tuna fish, fresh and smoked salmon, black tea, green tea, and black coffee.

Step 9. The following foods should not be consumed during the 30-day parasite treatment program; avoid all milk products, this includes cheese, yogurt, and butter. In addition, avoid all sugary foods and drinks, avoid diet sodas and or sweeteners of any kind. Primarily for the next 30 days you will be on a very restrictive low-carb diet, like a keto diet. You may lose approximately ten or more pounds within 30 days. Think of it this way, for parasites to live and thrive, they need a substantial amount of carbohydrates, and in order to eliminate the parasites, we must hold on to a strict low-carb diet during the 30 days parasite cleansing.

Step 10: Taking into consideration the 30-days of toxicity from antibiotics – you may feel tired and nauseated. A strict low-carb diet and fasting periods will be a challenge for most. Considering all it takes; this may explain the reason many individuals have a difficult time in eliminating parasites. There are cases where individuals have spent several years trying to cleanse themselves of parasites; this manual provides people a complete system and challenging 30-day parasite cleansing approach.

Step 11. During the 30-days parasite treatment plan, it is important for fasting, this includes 14 to 18 hours intermittent fasting and one of two days a week with 24 hour fasting periods. During the fasting, one can drink as much green or black tea, with some black coffee to keep you alert and awake if needed. Also, ensure you are drinking very clean filtered water, such as available at refill machines at Wholefoods Market, in order to eliminate the possibility of reinfections from the same and or any other parasites.

Step 12. After your 30-day parasite treatment plan, a few lab tests help diagnose parasitic diseases and other noninfectious causes of gastrointestinal symptoms: Stool (fecal) exam. This test looks for parasites or their eggs. Your doctor might give you a special container with preservative fluid for your stool samples.

Step 13. If the diagnose parasitic stool (fecal) exam comes back Negative – it is recommended you wait for an entire month before being tested again. This is important to allow for at least 30 days in order to find out if the parasites persist. Conduct the parasitic stool (fecal) exam for the next three months, every month in order you have been cleared of parasites. A fecal (stool) exam, also called an ova and parasite test (O&P). Good Luck! Do contact the author for comments and or recommendations that should be included in this book.

DAY 1

Prescription: Metronidazole (Flagyl) – 250 mg tablets each. Take 3 tablets by mouth three times daily, total 750 mg, for 30 days.

Essential Oils:
Clove Essential Oil (Organic if Available) 4 ounces
Oregano Oil, Wild – 4 ounces

Olive Oil (Organic) 32 ounces

Green Tea
Black Tea
Black Coffee
Peppermint tea

Mix ½ ounces clove oil and ½ ounces of oregano oil in 32 ounces clean filtered water.

1. Drink entire bottle of the mixture clove, oregano, and water within 8 hours, sipping every 30 minutes.
2. Metronidazole (Flagyl) – 250 mg tablets – 3 times a day.
3. Morning have a few cups of black tea
4. Afternoon a small meal of salad and fish
5. Green tea or coffee drinks as much as you want
6. Dinner onion, garlic, fish, and green vegetables
7. Peppermint tea
8. Midnight meal tuna – sardines

Notes:

DAY 2

Prescription: Metronidazole (Flagyl) – 250 mg tablets each. Take 3 tablets by mouth three times daily, total 750 mg, for 30 days.
Essential Oils:
Clove Essential Oil (Organic if Available) 4 ounces
Oregano Oil, Wild – 4 ounces

Olive Oil (Organic) 32 ounces

Green Tea
Black Tea
Black Coffee
Peppermint tea

Mix ½ ounces clove oil and ½ ounces of oregano oil in Olive Oil (Organic) 32 ounces

1.   Mixture of ½ ounce clove, ½ ounce oregano, and olive oil (organic) 32 ounces within 8 hours, 3 spoonful's a day.
2.   Metronidazole (Flagyl) – 250 mg tablets – 3 times a day.
3.   Morning have a few cups of black tea
4.   Fast until 5 PM and then have a small meal of salad and fish
5.   Green tea or coffee drinks as much as you want
6.   Dinner onion, garlic, fish, and green vegetables
7.   Peppermint tea
8.   Midnight meal tuna – sardines - onions green

DAY 3

Prescription: Metronidazole (Flagyl) – 250 mg tablets each. Take 3 tablets by mouth three times daily, total 750 mg, for 30 days.
Essential Oils:
Clove Essential Oil (Organic if Available) 4 ounces
Oregano Oil, Wild – 4 ounces

Olive Oil (Organic) 32 ounces

Green Tea
Black Tea
Black Coffee
Peppermint tea

Mix ½ ounces clove oil and ½ ounces of oregano oil in Olive Oil (Organic) 32 ounces

1.	Mixture of ½ ounce clove, ½ ounce oregano, and olive oil (organic) 32 ounces within 8 hours, 3 spoonful's a day.
2.	Metronidazole (Flagyl) – 250 mg tablets – 3 times a day.
3.	Morning have a few cups of black tea
4.	Fast until 5 PM and then have a small meal of salad and fish
5.	Green tea or coffee drinks as much as you want
6.	Dinner onion, garlic, fish, and green vegetables
7.	Peppermint tea
8.	Midnight meal tuna – sardines - onions green

DAY 4

Prescription: Metronidazole (Flagyl) – 250 mg tablets each. Take 3 tablets by mouth three times daily, total 750 mg, for 30 days.
Essential Oils:
Clove Essential Oil (Organic if Available) 4 ounces
Oregano Oil, Wild – 4 ounces

Olive Oil (Organic) 32 ounces

Green Tea
Black Tea
Black Coffee
Peppermint tea

Mix ½ ounces clove oil and ½ ounces of oregano oil in Olive Oil (Organic) 32 ounces

1.   Mixture of ½ ounce clove, ½ ounce oregano, and olive oil (organic) 32 ounces within 8 hours, 3 spoonful's a day.
2.   Metronidazole (Flagyl) – 250 mg tablets – 3 times a day.
3.   Morning have a few cups of black tea
4.   Fast until 5 PM and then have a small meal of salad and fish
5.   Green tea or coffee drinks as much as you want
6.   Dinner onion, garlic, fish, and green vegetables
7.   Peppermint tea
8.   Midnight meal tuna – sardines - onions green

DAY 5

Prescription: Metronidazole (Flagyl) – 250 mg tablets each. Take 3 tablets by mouth three times daily, total 750 mg, for 30 days.
Essential Oils:
Clove Essential Oil (Organic if Available) 4 ounces
Oregano Oil, Wild – 4 ounces

Olive Oil (Organic) 32 ounces

Green Tea
Black Tea
Black Coffee
Peppermint tea

Mix ½ ounces clove oil and ½ ounces of oregano oil in Olive Oil (Organic) 32 ounces

1.   Mixture of ½ ounce clove, ½ ounce oregano, and olive oil (organic) 32 ounces within 8 hours, 3 spoonful's a day.
2.   Metronidazole (Flagyl) – 250 mg tablets – 3 times a day.
3.   Morning have a few cups of black tea
4.   Fast until 10 PM and then have a small meal of salad and fish
5.   Green tea or coffee drinks as much as you want
6.   Dinner onion, garlic, fish, and green vegetables
7.   Peppermint tea
8.   Midnight meal tuna – sardines - onions green

DAY 6

Prescription: Metronidazole (Flagyl) – 250 mg tablets each. Take 3 tablets by mouth three times daily, total 750 mg, for 30 days.
Essential Oils:
Clove Essential Oil (Organic if Available) 4 ounces
Oregano Oil, Wild – 4 ounces

Olive Oil (Organic) 32 ounces

Green Tea
Black Tea
Black Coffee
Peppermint tea

Mix ½ ounces clove oil and ½ ounces of oregano oil in Olive Oil (Organic) 32 ounces

1.   Mixture of ½ ounce clove, ½ ounce oregano, and olive oil (organic) 32 ounces within 8 hours, 3 spoonful's a day.
2.   Metronidazole (Flagyl) – 250 mg tablets – 3 times a day.
3.   Morning have a few cups of black tea
4.   Fast until 5 PM and then have a small meal of salad and fish
5.   Green tea or coffee drinks as much as you want
6.   Dinner onion, garlic, fish, and green vegetables
7.   Peppermint tea
8.   Midnight meal tuna – sardines - onions green

DAY 7

Prescription: Metronidazole (Flagyl) – 250 mg tablets each. Take 3 tablets by mouth three times daily, total 750 mg, for 30 days.
Essential Oils:
Clove Essential Oil (Organic if Available) 4 ounces
Oregano Oil, Wild – 4 ounces

Olive Oil (Organic) 32 ounces

Green Tea
Black Tea
Black Coffee
Peppermint tea

Mix ½ ounces clove oil and ½ ounces of oregano oil in Olive Oil (Organic) 32 ounces

1.   Mixture of ½ ounce clove, ½ ounce oregano, and olive oil (organic) 32 ounces, 3 spoonful's a day.
2.   Metronidazole (Flagyl) – 250 mg tablets – 3 times a day.
3.   Morning have a few cups of black tea
4.   Fast until 5 PM and then have a small meal of salad and fish
5.   Green tea or coffee drinks as much as you want
6.   Dinner onion, garlic, fish, and green vegetables
7.   Peppermint tea
8.   Midnight meal tuna – sardines - onions green

DAY 8

Prescription: Metronidazole (Flagyl) – 250 mg tablets each. Take 3 tablets by mouth three times daily, total 750 mg, for 30 days.
Essential Oils:
Clove Essential Oil (Organic if Available) 4 ounces
Oregano Oil, Wild – 4 ounces

Olive Oil (Organic) 32 ounces

Green Tea
Black Tea
Black Coffee
Peppermint tea

Mix ½ ounces clove oil and ½ ounces of oregano oil in Olive Oil (Organic) 32 ounces

1.   Mixture of ½ ounce clove, ½ ounce oregano, and olive oil (organic) 32 ounces, 3 spoonful's a day.
2.   Metronidazole (Flagyl) – 250 mg tablets – 3 times a day.
3.   Morning have a few cups of black tea
4.   Fast until 10 PM and then have a small meal of salad and fish
5.   Green tea or coffee drinks as much as you want
6.   Dinner onion, garlic, fish, and green vegetables
7.   Peppermint tea
8.   Midnight meal tuna – sardines - onions green

Notes:

DAY 9

Prescription: Metronidazole (Flagyl) – 250 mg tablets each. Take 3 tablets by mouth three times daily, total 750 mg, for 30 days.
Essential Oils:
Clove Essential Oil (Organic if Available) 4 ounces
Oregano Oil, Wild – 4 ounces

Olive Oil (Organic) 32 ounces

Green Tea
Black Tea
Black Coffee
Peppermint tea

Mix ½ ounces clove oil and ½ ounces of oregano oil in Olive Oil (Organic) 32 ounces

1.	Mixture of ½ ounce clove, ½ ounce oregano, and olive oil (organic) 32 ounces, 3 spoonful's a day.
2.	Metronidazole (Flagyl) – 250 mg tablets – 3 times a day.
3.	Morning have a few cups of black tea
4.	Fast until 5 PM and then have a small meal of salad and fish
5.	Green tea or coffee drinks as much as you want
6.	Dinner onion, garlic, fish, and green vegetables
7.	Peppermint tea
8.	Midnight meal tuna – sardines - onions green

Notes:

DAY 10

Prescription: Metronidazole (Flagyl) – 250 mg tablets each. Take 3 tablets by mouth three times daily, total 750 mg, for 30 days.
Essential Oils:
Clove Essential Oil (Organic if Available) 4 ounces
Oregano Oil, Wild – 4 ounces

Olive Oil (Organic) 32 ounces

Green Tea
Black Tea
Black Coffee
Peppermint tea

Mix ½ ounces clove oil and ½ ounces of oregano oil in Olive Oil (Organic) 32 ounces

1.   Mixture of ½ ounce clove, ½ ounce oregano, and olive oil (organic) 32 ounces, 3 spoonful's a day.
2.   Metronidazole (Flagyl) – 250 mg tablets – 3 times a day.
3.   Morning have a few cups of black tea
4.   Fast until 5 PM and then have a small meal of salad and fish
5.   Green tea or coffee drinks as much as you want
6.   Dinner onion, garlic, fish, and green vegetables
7.   Peppermint tea
8.   Midnight meal tuna – sardines - onions green

Notes:

DAY 11

Prescription: Metronidazole (Flagyl) – 250 mg tablets each. Take 3 tablets by mouth three times daily, total 750 mg, for 30 days.
Essential Oils:
Clove Essential Oil (Organic if Available) 4 ounces
Oregano Oil, Wild – 4 ounces

Olive Oil (Organic) 32 ounces

Green Tea
Black Tea
Black Coffee
Peppermint tea

Mix ½ ounces clove oil and ½ ounces of oregano oil in Olive Oil (Organic) 32 ounces

1.   Mixture of ½ ounce clove, ½ ounce oregano, and olive oil (organic) 32 ounces, 3 spoonful's a day.
2.   Metronidazole (Flagyl) – 250 mg tablets – 3 times a day.
3.   Morning have a few cups of black tea
4.   Fast until 10 PM and then have a small meal of salad and fish
5.   Green tea or coffee drinks as much as you want
6.   Dinner onion, garlic, fish, and green vegetables
7.   Peppermint tea
8.   Midnight meal tuna – sardines - onions green

Notes:

DAY 12

Prescription: Metronidazole (Flagyl) – 250 mg tablets each. Take 3 tablets by mouth three times daily, total 750 mg, for 30 days.
Essential Oils:
Clove Essential Oil (Organic if Available) 4 ounces
Oregano Oil, Wild – 4 ounces

Olive Oil (Organic) 32 ounces

Green Tea
Black Tea
Black Coffee
Peppermint tea

Mix ½ ounces clove oil and ½ ounces of oregano oil in Olive Oil (Organic) 32 ounces

1.   Mixture of ½ ounce clove, ½ ounce oregano, and olive oil (organic) 32 ounces, 3 spoonful's a day.
2.   Metronidazole (Flagyl) – 250 mg tablets – 3 times a day.
3.   Morning have a few cups of black tea
4.   Fast until 5 PM and then have a small meal of salad and fish
5.   Green tea or coffee drinks as much as you want
6.   Dinner onion, garlic, fish, and green vegetables
7.   Peppermint tea
8.   Midnight meal tuna – sardines - onions green

Notes:

DAY 13

Prescription: Metronidazole (Flagyl) – 250 mg tablets each. Take 3 tablets by mouth three times daily, total 750 mg, for 30 days.
Essential Oils:
Clove Essential Oil (Organic if Available) 4 ounces
Oregano Oil, Wild – 4 ounces

Olive Oil (Organic) 32 ounces

Green Tea
Black Tea
Black Coffee
Peppermint tea

Mix ½ ounces clove oil and ½ ounces of oregano oil in Olive Oil (Organic) 32 ounces

1.   Mixture of ½ ounce clove, ½ ounce oregano, and olive oil (organic) 32 ounces, 3 spoonful's a day.
2.   Metronidazole (Flagyl) – 250 mg tablets – 3 times a day.
3.   Morning have a few cups of black tea
4.   Fast until 5 PM and then have a small meal of salad and fish
5.   Green tea or coffee drinks as much as you want
6.   Dinner onion, garlic, fish, and green vegetables
7.   Peppermint tea
8.   Midnight meal tuna – sardines - onions green

Notes:

DAY 14

Prescription: Metronidazole (Flagyl) – 250 mg tablets each. Take 3 tablets by mouth three times daily, total 750 mg, for 30 days.
Essential Oils:
Clove Essential Oil (Organic if Available) 4 ounces
Oregano Oil, Wild – 4 ounces

Olive Oil (Organic) 32 ounces

Green Tea
Black Tea
Black Coffee
Peppermint tea

Mix ½ ounces clove oil and ½ ounces of oregano oil in Olive Oil (Organic) 32 ounces

1.   Mixture of ½ ounce clove, ½ ounce oregano, and olive oil (organic) 32 ounces, 3 spoonful's a day.
2.   Metronidazole (Flagyl) – 250 mg tablets – 3 times a day.
3.   Morning have a few cups of black tea
4.   Fast until 5 PM and then have a small meal of salad and fish
5.   Green tea or coffee drinks as much as you want
6.   Dinner onion, garlic, fish, and green vegetables
7.   Peppermint tea
8.   Midnight meal tuna – sardines - onions green

Notes:

DAY 15

Prescription: Metronidazole (Flagyl) – 250 mg tablets each. Take 3 tablets by mouth three times daily, total 750 mg, for 30 days.
Essential Oils:
Clove Essential Oil (Organic if Available) 4 ounces
Oregano Oil, Wild – 4 ounces

Olive Oil (Organic) 32 ounces

Green Tea
Black Tea
Black Coffee
Peppermint tea

Mix ½ ounces clove oil and ½ ounces of oregano oil in Olive Oil (Organic) 32 ounces

1.	Mixture of ½ ounce clove, ½ ounce oregano, and olive oil (organic) 32 ounces, 3 spoonful's a day.
2.	Metronidazole (Flagyl) – 250 mg tablets – 3 times a day.
3.	Morning have a few cups of black tea
4.	Fast until 10 PM and then have a small meal of salad and fish
5.	Green tea or coffee drinks as much as you want
6.	Dinner onion, garlic, fish, and green vegetables
7.	Peppermint tea
8.	Midnight meal tuna – sardines - onions green

Notes:

DAY 16

Prescription: Metronidazole (Flagyl) – 250 mg tablets each. Take 3 tablets by mouth three times daily, total 750 mg, for 30 days.
Essential Oils:
Clove Essential Oil (Organic if Available) 4 ounces
Oregano Oil, Wild – 4 ounces

Olive Oil (Organic) 32 ounces

Green Tea
Black Tea
Black Coffee
Peppermint tea

Mix ½ ounces clove oil and ½ ounces of oregano oil in 32 ounces clean filtered water.

1.   Drink entire bottle of the mixture clove, oregano, and water within 8 hours, sipping every 30 minutes.
2.   Metronidazole (Flagyl) – 250 mg tablets – 3 times a day.
3.   Morning have a few cups of black tea
4.   Afternoon a small meal of salad and fish
5.   Green tea or coffee drinks as much as you want
6.   Dinner onion, garlic, fish, and green vegetables
7.   Peppermint tea
8.   Midnight meal tuna – sardines

Notes:

DAY 17

Prescription: Metronidazole (Flagyl) – 250 mg tablets each. Take 3 tablets by mouth three times daily, total 750 mg, for 30 days.
Essential Oils:
Clove Essential Oil (Organic if Available) 4 ounces
Oregano Oil, Wild – 4 ounces

Olive Oil (Organic) 32 ounces

Green Tea
Black Tea
Black Coffee
Peppermint tea

Mix ½ ounces clove oil and ½ ounces of oregano oil in 32 ounces clean filtered water.

1.   Drink entire bottle of the mixture clove, oregano, and water within 8 hours, sipping every 30 minutes.
2.   Metronidazole (Flagyl) – 250 mg tablets – 3 times a day.
3.   Morning have a few cups of black tea
4.   Afternoon a small meal of salad and fish
5.   Green tea or coffee drinks as much as you want
6.   Dinner onion, garlic, fish, and green vegetables
7.   Peppermint tea
8.   Midnight meal tuna – sardines

Notes:

DAY 18

Prescription: Metronidazole (Flagyl) – 250 mg tablets each. Take 3 tablets by mouth three times daily, total 750 mg, for 30 days.
Essential Oils:
Clove Essential Oil (Organic if Available) 4 ounces
Oregano Oil, Wild – 4 ounces

Olive Oil (Organic) 32 ounces

Green Tea
Black Tea
Black Coffee
Peppermint tea

Mix ½ ounces clove oil and ½ ounces of oregano oil in 32 ounces clean filtered water.

1.   Drink entire bottle of the mixture clove, oregano, and water within 8 hours, sipping every 30 minutes.
2.   Metronidazole (Flagyl) – 250 mg tablets – 3 times a day.
3.   Morning have a few cups of black tea
4.   Afternoon a small meal of salad and fish
5.   Green tea or coffee drinks as much as you want
6.   Dinner onion, garlic, fish, and green vegetables
7.   Peppermint tea
8.   Midnight meal tuna – sardines

Notes:

DAY 19

Prescription: Metronidazole (Flagyl) – 250 mg tablets each. Take 3 tablets by mouth three times daily, total 750 mg, for 30 days.
Essential Oils:
Clove Essential Oil (Organic if Available) 4 ounces
Oregano Oil, Wild – 4 ounces

Olive Oil (Organic) 32 ounces

Green Tea
Black Tea
Black Coffee
Peppermint tea

Mix ½ ounces clove oil and ½ ounces of oregano oil in Olive Oil (Organic) 32 ounces

1.   Mixture of ½ ounce clove, ½ ounce oregano, and olive oil (organic) 32 ounces, 3 spoonful's a day.
2.   Metronidazole (Flagyl) – 250 mg tablets – 3 times a day.
3.   Morning have a few cups of black tea
4.   Fast until 5 PM and then have a small meal of salad and fish
5.   Green tea or coffee drinks as much as you want
6.   Dinner onion, garlic, fish, and green vegetables
7.   Peppermint tea
8.   Midnight meal tuna – sardines - onions green

Notes:

DAY 20

Prescription: Metronidazole (Flagyl) – 250 mg tablets each. Take 3 tablets by mouth three times daily, total 750 mg, for 30 days.
Essential Oils:
Clove Essential Oil (Organic if Available) 4 ounces
Oregano Oil, Wild – 4 ounces

Olive Oil (Organic) 32 ounces

Green Tea
Black Tea
Black Coffee
Peppermint tea

Mix ½ ounces clove oil and ½ ounces of oregano oil in Olive Oil (Organic) 32 ounces

1.   Mixture of ½ ounce clove, ½ ounce oregano, and olive oil (organic) 32 ounces, 3 spoonful's a day.
2.   Metronidazole (Flagyl) – 250 mg tablets – 3 times a day.
3.   Morning have a few cups of black tea
4.   Fast until 5 PM and then have a small meal of salad and fish
5.   Green tea or coffee drinks as much as you want
6.   Dinner onion, garlic, fish, and green vegetables
7.   Peppermint tea
8.   Midnight meal tuna – sardines - onions green

Notes:

DAY 21

Prescription: Metronidazole (Flagyl) – 250 mg tablets each. Take 3 tablets by mouth three times daily, total 750 mg, for 30 days.
Essential Oils:
Clove Essential Oil (Organic if Available) 4 ounces
Oregano Oil, Wild – 4 ounces

Olive Oil (Organic) 32 ounces

Green Tea
Black Tea
Black Coffee
Peppermint tea

Mix ½ ounces clove oil and ½ ounces of oregano oil in Olive Oil (Organic) 32 ounces

1.   Mixture of ½ ounce clove, ½ ounce oregano, and olive oil (organic) 32 ounces, 3 spoonful's a day.
2.   Metronidazole (Flagyl) – 250 mg tablets – 3 times a day.
3.   Morning have a few cups of black tea
4.   Fast until 5 PM and then have a small meal of salad and fish
5.   Green tea or coffee drinks as much as you want
6.   Dinner onion, garlic, fish, and green vegetables
7.   Peppermint tea
8.   Midnight meal tuna – sardines - onions green

Notes:

DAY 22

Prescription: Metronidazole (Flagyl) – 250 mg tablets each. Take 3 tablets by mouth three times daily, total 750 mg, for 30 days.
Essential Oils:
Clove Essential Oil (Organic if Available) 4 ounces
Oregano Oil, Wild – 4 ounces

Olive Oil (Organic) 32 ounces

Green Tea
Black Tea
Black Coffee
Peppermint tea

Mix ½ ounces clove oil and ½ ounces of oregano oil in Olive Oil (Organic) 32 ounces

1.   Mixture of ½ ounce clove, ½ ounce oregano, and olive oil (organic) 32 ounces, 3 spoonful's a day.
2.   Metronidazole (Flagyl) – 250 mg tablets – 3 times a day.
3.   Morning have a few cups of black tea
4.   Fast until 5 PM and then have a small meal of salad and fish
5.   Green tea or coffee drinks as much as you want
6.   Dinner onion, garlic, fish, and green vegetables
7.   Peppermint tea
8.   Midnight meal tuna – sardines - onions green

Notes:

DAY 23

Prescription: Metronidazole (Flagyl) – 250 mg tablets each. Take 3 tablets by mouth three times daily, total 750 mg, for 30 days.
Essential Oils:
Clove Essential Oil (Organic if Available) 4 ounces
Oregano Oil, Wild – 4 ounces

Olive Oil (Organic) 32 ounces

Green Tea
Black Tea
Black Coffee
Peppermint tea

Mix ½ ounces clove oil and ½ ounces of oregano oil in Olive Oil (Organic) 32 ounces

1.   Mixture of ½ ounce clove, ½ ounce oregano, and olive oil (organic) 32 ounces, 3 spoonful's a day.
2.   Metronidazole (Flagyl) – 250 mg tablets – 3 times a day.
3.   Morning have a few cups of black tea
4.   Fast until 5 PM and then have a small meal of salad and fish
5.   Green tea or coffee drinks as much as you want
6.   Dinner onion, garlic, fish, and green vegetables
7.   Peppermint tea
8.   Midnight meal tuna – sardines - onions green

Notes:

DAY 24

Prescription: Metronidazole (Flagyl) – 250 mg tablets each. Take 3 tablets by mouth three times daily, total 750 mg, for 30 days.
Essential Oils:
Clove Essential Oil (Organic if Available) 4 ounces
Oregano Oil, Wild – 4 ounces

Olive Oil (Organic) 32 ounces

Green Tea
Black Tea
Black Coffee
Peppermint tea

Mix ½ ounces clove oil and ½ ounces of oregano oil in Olive Oil (Organic) 32 ounces

1.   Mixture of ½ ounce clove, ½ ounce oregano, and olive oil (organic) 32 ounces, 3 spoonful's a day.
2.   Metronidazole (Flagyl) – 250 mg tablets – 3 times a day.
3.   Morning have a few cups of black tea
4.   Fast until 5 PM and then have a small meal of salad and fish
5.   Green tea or coffee drinks as much as you want
6.   Dinner onion, garlic, fish, and green vegetables
7.   Peppermint tea
8.   Midnight meal tuna – sardines - onions green

Notes:

DAY 25

Prescription: Metronidazole (Flagyl) – 250 mg tablets each. Take 3 tablets by mouth three times daily, total 750 mg, for 30 days.
Essential Oils:
Clove Essential Oil (Organic if Available) 4 ounces
Oregano Oil, Wild – 4 ounces

Olive Oil (Organic) 32 ounces

Green Tea
Black Tea
Black Coffee
Peppermint tea

Mix ½ ounces clove oil and ½ ounces of oregano oil in Olive Oil (Organic) 32 ounces

1.	Mixture of ½ ounce clove, ½ ounce oregano, and olive oil (organic) 32 ounces, 3 spoonful's a day.
2.	Metronidazole (Flagyl) – 250 mg tablets – 3 times a day.
3.	Morning have a few cups of black tea
4.	Fast until 5 PM and then have a small meal of salad and fish
5.	Green tea or coffee drinks as much as you want
6.	Dinner onion, garlic, fish, and green vegetables
7.	Peppermint tea
8.	Midnight meal tuna – sardines - onions green

Notes:

DAY 26

Prescription: Metronidazole (Flagyl) – 250 mg tablets each. Take 3 tablets by mouth three times daily, total 750 mg, for 30 days.
Essential Oils:
Clove Essential Oil (Organic if Available) 4 ounces
Oregano Oil, Wild – 4 ounces

Olive Oil (Organic) 32 ounces

Green Tea
Black Tea
Black Coffee
Peppermint tea

Mix ½ ounces clove oil and ½ ounces of oregano oil in Olive Oil (Organic) 32 ounces

1.   Mixture of ½ ounce clove, ½ ounce oregano, and olive oil (organic) 32 ounces, 3 spoonful's a day.
2.   Metronidazole (Flagyl) – 250 mg tablets – 3 times a day.
3.   Morning have a few cups of black tea
4.   Fast until 5 PM and then have a small meal of salad and fish
5.   Green tea or coffee drinks as much as you want
6.   Dinner onion, garlic, fish, and green vegetables
7.   Peppermint tea
8.   Midnight meal tuna – sardines - onions green

Notes:

DAY 27

Prescription: Metronidazole (Flagyl) – 250 mg tablets each. Take 3 tablets by mouth three times daily, total 750 mg, for 30 days.
Essential Oils:
Clove Essential Oil (Organic if Available) 4 ounces
Oregano Oil, Wild – 4 ounces

Olive Oil (Organic) 32 ounces

Green Tea
Black Tea
Black Coffee
Peppermint tea

Mix ½ ounces clove oil and ½ ounces of oregano oil in 32 ounces clean filtered water.

1.   Drink entire bottle of the mixture clove, oregano, and water within 8 hours, sipping every 30 minutes.
2.   Metronidazole (Flagyl) – 250 mg tablets – 3 times a day.
3.   Morning have a few cups of black tea
4.   Afternoon a small meal of salad and fish
5.   Green tea or coffee drinks as much as you want
6.   Dinner onion, garlic, fish, and green vegetables
7.   Peppermint tea
8.   Midnight meal tuna – sardines

Notes:

DAY 28

Prescription: Metronidazole (Flagyl) – 250 mg tablets each. Take 3 tablets by mouth three times daily, total 750 mg, for 30 days.
Essential Oils:
Clove Essential Oil (Organic if Available) 4 ounces
Oregano Oil, Wild – 4 ounces

Olive Oil (Organic) 32 ounces

Green Tea
Black Tea
Black Coffee
Peppermint tea

Mix ½ ounces clove oil and ½ ounces of oregano oil in 32 ounces clean filtered water.

1.   Drink entire bottle of the mixture clove, oregano, and water within 8 hours, sipping every 30 minutes.
2.   Metronidazole (Flagyl) – 250 mg tablets – 3 times a day.
3.   Morning have a few cups of black tea
4.   Afternoon a small meal of salad and fish
5.   Green tea or coffee drinks as much as you want
6.   Dinner onion, garlic, fish, and green vegetables
7.   Peppermint tea
8.   Midnight meal tuna – sardines

Notes:

DAY 29

Prescription: Metronidazole (Flagyl) – 250 mg tablets each. Take 3 tablets by mouth three times daily, total 750 mg, for 30 days.
Essential Oils:
Clove Essential Oil (Organic if Available) 4 ounces
Oregano Oil, Wild – 4 ounces

Olive Oil (Organic) 32 ounces

Green Tea
Black Tea
Black Coffee
Peppermint tea

Mix ½ ounces clove oil and ½ ounces of oregano oil in Olive Oil (Organic) 32 ounces

1. Mixture of ½ ounce clove, ½ ounce oregano, and olive oil (organic) 32 ounces, 3 spoonful's a day.
2. Metronidazole (Flagyl) – 250 mg tablets – 3 times a day.
3. Morning have a few cups of black tea
4. Fast until 5 PM and then have a small meal of salad and fish
5. Green tea or coffee drinks as much as you want
6. Dinner onion, garlic, fish, and green vegetables
7. Peppermint tea
8. Midnight meal tuna – sardines - onions green

Notes:

DAY 30

Prescription: Metronidazole (Flagyl) – 250 mg tablets each. Take 3 tablets by mouth three times daily, total 750 mg, for 30 days.

Essential Oils:

Clove Essential Oil (Organic if Available) 4 ounces

Oregano Oil, Wild – 4 ounces

Olive Oil (Organic) 32 ounces

Green Tea

Black Tea

Black Coffee

Peppermint tea

Mix ½ ounces clove oil and ½ ounces of oregano oil in Olive Oil (Organic) 32 ounces

1.   Mixture of ½ ounce clove, ½ ounce oregano, and olive oil (organic) 32 ounces, 3 spoonful's a day.
2.   Metronidazole (Flagyl) – 250 mg tablets – 3 times a day.
3.   Morning have a few cups of black tea
4.   Fast until 5 PM and then have a small meal of salad and fish
5.   Green tea or coffee drinks as much as you want
6.   Dinner onion, garlic, fish, and green vegetables
7.   Peppermint tea
8.   Midnight meal tuna – sardines - onions green

Notes:

Notes:

Notes:

Notes:

Parasites

About Parasites

A parasite is an organism that lives on or in a host organism and gets its food from or at the expense of its host. There are three main classes of parasites that can cause disease in humans: protozoa, helminths, and ectoparasites.

Parasitic infections are typically associated with poor and often marginalized communities in low-income countries. However, these infections are also present in the United States.

The neglected parasitic infections (NPIs) are a group of five parasitic diseases that have been targeted by the CDC as priorities for public health action based on the

• Number of people infected

• Severity of the illnesses

• Ability to prevent and treat them

These infections are considered neglected because relatively little attention has been devoted to their surveillance, prevention, and/or treatment.

Anyone, regardless of race or economic status, can become infected although minorities, immigrants, and people living in poor or disadvantaged communities appear to be most at risk.

CDC is working to protect people from these health threats by

• Increasing awareness among physicians and the public

• Synthesizing the existing data to help better understand these infections

• Improving diagnostic testing

• Advising on treatment, including distributing otherwise unavailable drugs for certain infections (Chagas disease)

Protozoa

Protozoa are microscopic, one-celled organisms that can be free-living or parasitic in nature. They can multiply in humans, which contributes to their survival and permits serious infections to develop from just a single organism. Transmission of protozoa that live in a human's intestine to another human typically occurs through a fecal-oral route (for example, contaminated food or water or person-to-person contact). Protozoa that live in the blood or tissue of humans are transmitted to other humans by an arthropod vector (for example, through the bite of a mosquito or sand fly).

The protozoa that are infectious to humans can be classified into four groups based on their mode of movement:
Sarcodina – the ameba, e.g., Entamoeba Mastigophora – the flagellates, e.g., Giardia, Leishmania Ciliophora – the ciliates, e.g., Balantidium Sporozoa – organisms whose adult stage is not motile e.g., Plasmodium, Cryptosporidium

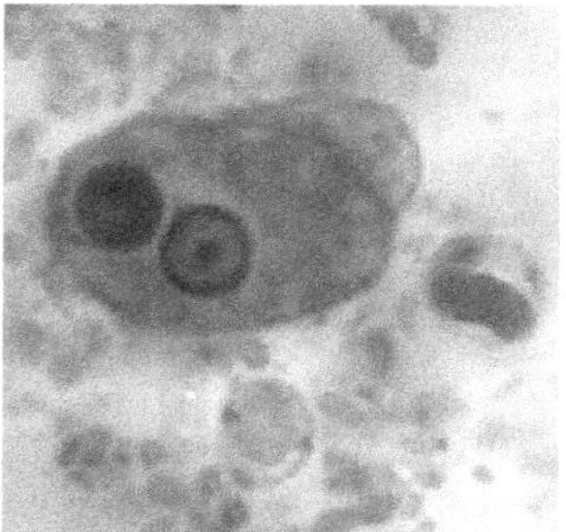

Entamoeba histolytica is a protozoan. A microscope is necessary to view this parasite. Credit CDC.

Helminths

Helminths are large, multicellular organisms that are generally visible to the naked eye in their adult stages. Like protozoa, helminths can be either free-living or parasitic in nature. In their adult form, helminths cannot multiply in humans. There are three main groups of helminths (derived from the Greek word for worms) that are human parasites:

Flatworms (platyhelminths) – these include the trematodes (flukes) and cestodes (tapeworms).

Thorny-headed worms (acanthocephalins) – the adult forms of these worms reside in the gastrointestinal tract. The acanthocephala are thought to be intermediate between the cestodes and nematodes.

Roundworms (nematodes) – the adult forms of these worms can reside in the gastrointestinal tract, blood, lymphatic system or subcutaneous tissues. Alternatively, the immature (larval) states can cause disease through their infection of various body tissues. Some consider the helminths to also include the segmented worms (annelids)—the only ones important medically are the leeches. Of note, these organisms are not typically considered parasites.

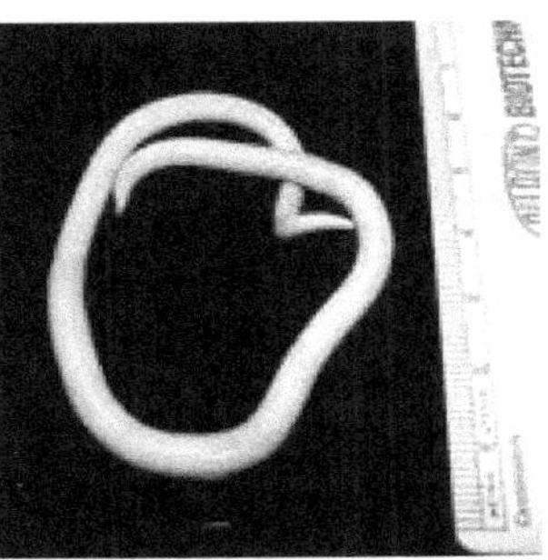

An adult Ascaris lumbriocoides worm. They can range from 15 to 35 cm. Credit CDC.

Ectoparasites

Although the term ectoparasites can broadly include blood-sucking arthropods such as mosquitoes (because they are dependent on a blood meal from a human host for their survival), this term is generally used more narrowly to refer to organisms such as ticks, fleas, lice, and mites that attach or burrow into the skin and remain there for relatively long periods of time (e.g., weeks to months). Arthropods are important in causing diseases in their own right, but are even more important as vectors, or transmitters, of many different pathogens that in turn cause tremendous morbidity and mortality from the diseases they cause.

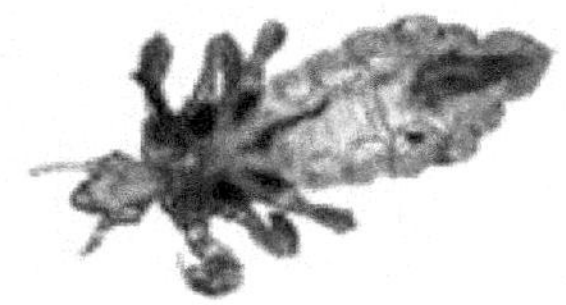

An adult louse. Acutal size is about as big as a sesame seed. Credit CDC.

Parasitic Infections

Parasitic infections cause a tremendous burden of disease in both the tropics and subtropics as well as in more temperate climates. Of all parasitic diseases, malaria causes the most deaths globally. Malaria kills approximately 660,000 people each year, most of them young children in sub-Saharan Africa.

The Neglected Tropical Diseases (NTDs), which have suffered from a lack of attention by the public health community, include parasitic diseases such as lymphatic filariasis, onchocerciasis, and Guinea worm disease. The NTDs affect more than 1 billion people—one-sixth of the world's population—largely in rural areas of low-income countries. These diseases extract a large toll on endemic populations, including lost ability to attend school or work, retardation of growth in children, impairment of cognitive skills and development in young children, and the serious economic burden placed on entire countries.

However, parasitic infections also affect persons living in developed countries, including the United States.

Diagnosis of Parasitic Diseases

How are parasitic diseases diagnosed?

Many kinds of lab tests are available to diagnose parasitic diseases. The kind of test(s) your health care provider will order will be based on your signs and symptoms, any other medical conditions you may have, and your travel history. Diagnosis may be difficult, so your health care provider may order more than one kind of test.

What kinds of tests are used to diagnose parasitic diseases?

See below for a list of some commonly used tests your health care provider may order.

A fecal (stool) exam, also called an ova and parasite test (O&P)

This test is used to find parasites that cause diarrhea, loose or watery stools, cramping, flatulence (gas) and other abdominal illness. CDC recommends that three or more stool samples, collected on separate days, be examined. This test looks for ova (eggs) or the parasite. Your health care provider may instruct you to put your stool specimens into special containers with preservative fluid. Specimens not collected in a preservative fluid should be refrigerated, but not frozen, until delivered to the lab or the health care provider's office. Your health care provider may request that the lab use special stains or that special tests be performed to look for parasites not routinely screened for.

Endoscopy/Colonoscopy

Endoscopy is used to find parasites that cause diarrhea, loose or watery stools, cramping, flatulence (gas) and other abdominal illness. This test is used when stool exams do not reveal the cause of your diarrhea. This test is a procedure in which a tube is inserted into the mouth (endoscopy) or rectum (colonoscopy) so that the doctor, usually a gastroenterologist, can examine the intestine. This test looks for the parasite or other abnormalities that may be causing your signs and symptoms.

Blood tests

Some, but not all, parasitic infections can be detected by testing your blood. Blood tests look for a specific parasite infection; there is no blood test that will look for all parasitic infections. There are two general kinds of blood tests that your doctor may order:

Serology

This test is used to look for antibodies or for parasite antigens produced when the body is infected with a parasite and the immune system is trying to fight off the invader. This test is done by your health care provider taking a blood sample and sending it to a lab.

Blood smear

This test is used to look for parasites that are found in the blood. By looking at a blood smear under a microscope, parasitic diseases such as filariasis, malaria, or babesiosis, can be diagnosed. This test is done by placing a drop of blood on a microscope slide. The slide is then stained and examined under a microscope.

X-ray, Magnetic Resonance Imaging (MRI) scan, Computerized Axial Tomography scan (CAT)These tests are used to look for some parasitic diseases that may cause lesions in the organs.

Where should lab specimens be sent for testing?

Blood testing is done by a variety of labs. Your health care provider will decide where to send the blood samples to.

Diagnosis of any stool parasite may be difficult; by submitting several stool specimens, your chance of being diagnosed correctly is higher than by submitting just one sample. If you receive a negative lab report, your physician may choose to send another sample to a different lab for confirmation.

Is it true that labs in the United States cannot diagnose parasites?

No. Labs throughout the United States are qualified to diagnose parasitic infections. Some labs have more experience than others or use various tests for the same parasite. Therefore, your health care provider may have more than one lab look at a sample if the suspicion of a parasitic infection is strong.

Transmission of Parasitic Diseases

Animals (Zoonotic)

Pets can carry parasites and pass parasites to people. Proper handwashing can greatly reduce risk.

A zoonotic disease is a disease spread between animals and people. Zoonotic diseases can be caused by viruses, bacteria, parasites, and fungi. Some of these diseases are very common. For zoonotic diseases that are caused by parasites, the types of symptoms and signs can be different depending on the parasite and the person. Sometimes people with zoonotic infections can be very sick but some people have no symptoms and do not ever get sick. Other people may have symptoms such as diarrhea, muscle aches, and fever.

Foods can be the source for some zoonotic infection when animals such as cows and pigs are infected with parasites such as Cryptosporidium or Trichinella. People can acquire cryptosporidiosis if they accidentally swallow food or water that is contaminated by stool from infected animals.

For example, this can happen when orchards or water sources are near cow pastures and people consume the fruit without proper washing or drink untreated water. People can acquire trichinellosis by ingesting undercooked or raw meat from bear, boar, or domestic pigs that are infected with the Trichinella parasite.

Pets can carry and pass parasites to people.

Some dog and cat parasites can infect people. Young animals, such as puppies and kittens, are more likely to be infected with roundworms and hookworms.

Wild animals can also be infected with parasites that can infect people. For example, people can be infected by the raccoon parasite Baylisascaris if they accidentally swallow soil that is contaminated with infected raccoon feces.

Regular veterinary care will protect your pet and your family.

There are simple steps you can take to protect yourself and your family from zoonotic diseases caused by parasites.

Make sure your pet is under a veterinarian's care to help protect your pet and your family from possible parasite infections.

Practice the four Ps: Pick up Pet Poop Promptly, and dispose of properly. Be sure to wash your hands after handling pet waste.

Wash your hands frequently, especially after touching animals, and avoid contact with animal feces.

Follow proper food-handling procedures to reduce the risk of transmission from contaminated food.

For people with weakened immune systems, be especially careful of contact with animals that could transmit these infections.

Blood

Some parasites can be bloodborne. This means:

the parasite can be found in the bloodstream of infected people; and the parasite might be spread to other people through exposure to an infected person's blood (for example, by blood transfusion or by sharing needles or syringes contaminated with blood).

Examples of parasitic diseases that can be bloodborne include African trypanosomiasis, babesiosis, Chagas disease, leishmaniasis, malaria, and toxoplasmosis. In nature, many bloodborne parasites are spread by insects (vectors), so they are also referred to as vector-borne diseases. Toxoplasma gondii is not transmitted by an insect (vector).

In the United States, the risk for vector-borne transmission is very low for these parasites except for some Babesia species.

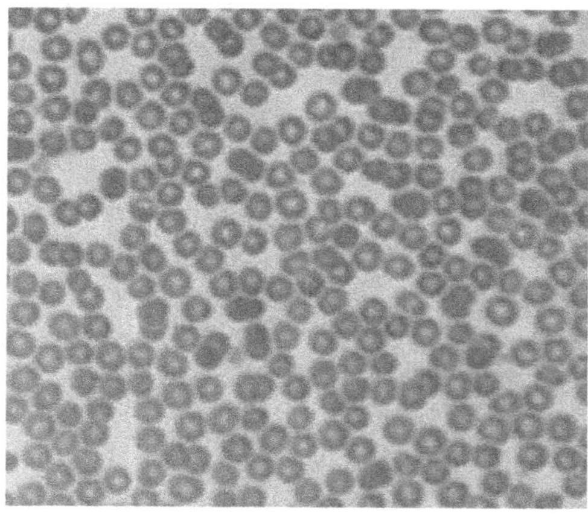

Microscopic red blood cells.

Blood Transfusions

Many factors affect whether parasites that can be found in the bloodstream might be spread by blood transfusion. Examples of some of the factors include:

how much of the parasite's life cycle is spent in the blood;
how many parasites might be found in the blood (in other words, the concentration or level of the parasite);
how long the parasite stays in the body, in treated and untreated people; and
how the parasite affects people. For example, if infected people feel sick, they might not want to donate blood, or they might be deferred (turned away).

Some parasites spend most or all of their life cycle in the bloodstream, such as Babesia and Plasmodium species. Parasites, such as Trypanosoma cruzi, might be found in the blood early in an infection (the acute phase) and then at much lower levels later (the chronic phase of infection). Other parasites only migrate (travel) through the blood to get to another part of the body.

There may be cases of transfusion-transmitted parasites that go undetected and unreported, but the risk for infection is very low compared with the number of blood transfusions. In the United States since 1980, there have been published reports of cases of transfusion-associated babesiosis (>150), malaria (~50), and Chagas disease (~5). Since 1965, there have been published reports of transfusion-associated toxoplasmosis (~4).

Blood Donor Screening

Potential blood donors are asked if they have had babesiosis or Chagas disease. If the answer is "yes," the person is deferred from donating blood.

Potential blood donors are also asked about their recent international travel. People who traveled to an are where malaria transmission occurs are deferred from donating blood for 1 year after their return to the United States.

Former residents of areas where malaria transmission occurs will be deferred for 3 years. People diagnosed with malaria cannot donate blood for 3 years after treatment, during which time they must have remained free of symptoms of malaria.

Donated blood is tested for a number of infectious agents. Currently, most of the U.S. blood supply is screened for Trypanosoma cruzi (the parasite that causes Chagas disease). If the results are positive, the blood center will try to notify the donor. People who test positive should consult a health care provider. Health care providers may contact CDC for confirmatory testing and management information, including treatment.

Food

Numerous parasites can be transmitted by food including many protozoa and helminths. In the United States, the most common foodborne parasites are protozoa such as Cryptosporidium spp., Giardia intestinalis, Cyclospora cayetanensis, and Toxoplasma gondii; roundworms such as Trichinella spp. and Anisakis spp.; and tapeworms such as Diphyllobothrium spp. and Taenia spp.

Many of these organisms can also be transmitted by water, soil, or person-to-person contact. Occasionally in the U.S., but often in developing countries, a wide variety of helminthic roundworms, tapeworms, and flukes are transmitted in foods such as

undercooked fish, crabs, and mollusks.
undercooked meat; raw aquatic plants such as watercress.
raw vegetables that have been contaminated by human or animal feces.
Some foods are contaminated by food service workers who practice poor hygiene or who work in unsanitary facilities.

Symptoms of foodborne parasitic infections vary greatly depending on the type of parasite. Protozoa such as Cryptosporidium spp., Giardia intestinalis, and Cyclospora cayetanensis most commonly cause diarrhea and other gastrointestinal symptoms. Helminthic infections can cause abdominal pain, diarrhea, muscle pain, cough, skin lesions, malnutrition, weight loss, neurological and many other symptoms depending on the organism and burden of infection. Treatment is available for most of the foodborne parasitic organisms.

Insects

Triatomine bugs are the vectors for Chagas disease.

An insect that transmits a disease is known as a vector, and the disease is referred to as a vector-borne disease. Insects can act as mechanical vectors, meaning that the insect can carry an organism, but the insect is not essential to the organism's life cycle, such as when house flies carry organisms on the outside of their bodies that cause diarrhea in people. Insects can also serve as obligatory hosts where the disease-causing organism must undergo development before being transmitted (as in the case with malaria parasites).

Vector-borne transmission of disease can take place when the parasite enters the host through the saliva of the insect during a blood meal (for example, malaria and dengue), or from parasites in the feces of the insect that defecates immediately after a blood meal (for example, Chagas disease). Parasites transmitted by insects often circulate in the blood of the host, with the parasite residing in and damaging organs or other parts of the body.

n developing countries where insect control is less common, the frequency of diseases is usually greater than in areas with the resources to effectively reduce the populations of disease vector insects. In the United States, the risk for vector-borne transmission is very low for these parasites except for some Babesia species.

It is important to remember that while some species of insects are capable of transmitting disease, the majority of insects are beneficial to people and the environment.

Water

Parasites can live in natural water sources. When outdoors, treat your water before drinking it to avoid getting sick.

Water is an essential resource for life. Water is used by everyone, every day. Not only do all people need drinking water to survive, but water plays an important role in almost every aspect of our lives – from recreation to manufacturing computers to performing medical procedures. When water becomes contaminated by parasites, however, it can cause a variety of illnesses.

Globally, contaminated water is a serious problem that can cause severe pain, disability and even death. Common global water-related diseases caused by parasites include Guinea worm, schistosomiasis, amebiasis, cryptosporidiosis (Crypto), and giardiasis. People become infected with these diseases when they swallow or have contact with water that has been contaminated by certain parasites. For example, individuals drinking water contaminated with fecal matter containing the ameba Entamoeba histolytica can get amebic dysentery (amebiasis). An individual can get Guinea worm disease when they drink water that contains the parasite Dracunculus medinensis. If an infected person with an open Guinea worm wound enters a pond or well used for drinking water, they can spread the parasite into the water and continue the cycle of contamination and infection. Schistosomiasis can be spread when people swim in or have contact with freshwater lakes that are contaminated with Schistosoma parasites.

Americans traveling abroad should take the necessary precautions to protect themselves from waterborne illness if they plan on being in countries with unsafe drinking water or recreational water. Individuals spending time in the wilderness should also follow the appropriate steps to ensure the safety of their water.

Parasites are also a cause of waterborne disease in the United States. Both recreational water (water used for swimming and other activities) and drinking water can become contaminated with parasites and cause illness. Recreational water illnesses (RWIs) are diseases that are spread by swallowing, breathing, or having contact with contaminated water from swimming pools, hot tubs, lakes, rivers, or the ocean.

The most commonly reported RWI is diarrhea caused by parasites, such as Cryptosporidium and Giardia intestinalis. Giardia intestinalis is also a common parasite found in drinking water. Both Cryptosporidium and Giardia intestinalis are found in the fecal matter of an infected person or animal. These parasites can be spread when someone swallows' water that has been contaminated with fecal matter from an infected person or animal. Individuals with compromised immune systems who encounter these parasites can also be at greater risk for serious illness.

Proper sanitation and hygiene are also essential to preventing waterborne illness. Globally, CDC works to provide access to clean and safe water through a variety of programs and projects. In the United States, CDC educates the public on how to develop healthy swimming habits and protect their private well water from parasites.

Women

Infection with several parasites can lead to special consequences for women. Some examples are given below.

Infection with Toxoplasma gondii, a parasite found in undercooked meat, cat feces, soil, and untreated water can lead to severe brain and eye disorders in a fetus when a pregnant woman becomes newly infected.
Trichomonas vaginalis, a sexually transmitted parasite that can be passed between partners, can lead to vaginal infection and increase a woman's susceptibility to human immunodeficiency virus (HIV) infection.
Pregnant women in malaria-endemic countries are at increased risk for adverse effects of malaria infection (for example, miscarriage, low birth weight).

Children

Parasitic infection or infestation can occur in children of all ages. Infants, toddlers, and very young children in day care settings are at risk for the parasitic disease called giardiasis that causes diarrhea and is spread through contaminated feces. Pinworm infection (enterobiasis) also occurs among preschool and young school-age children. Both preschool and school-age children can become infested with head lice (pediculosis) or scabies, both of which are spread by close person-to-person contact as is common during childhood play.

Travel/Travelers

International travelers can be at risk for a variety of infectious and non-infectious diseases. Travelers may acquire parasitic illnesses:

through ingestion of contaminated food or water,
by vector-borne transmission, or
through person-to-person contact.

Contaminated food and drink are common sources for the introduction of infection into the body. The table below shows some of the more common parasitic infections that travelers can acquire from contaminated food and drink, as well as a few of the less common parasitic diseases that travelers are at risk for acquiring. The risk of acquiring these other protozoa and helminths varies greatly by region of the world and specific country. Many infectious diseases transmitted in food and water can also be acquired directly through the fecal-oral route.

Parasites — Acanthamoeba — Granulomatous Amebic Encephalitis (GAE); Keratitis

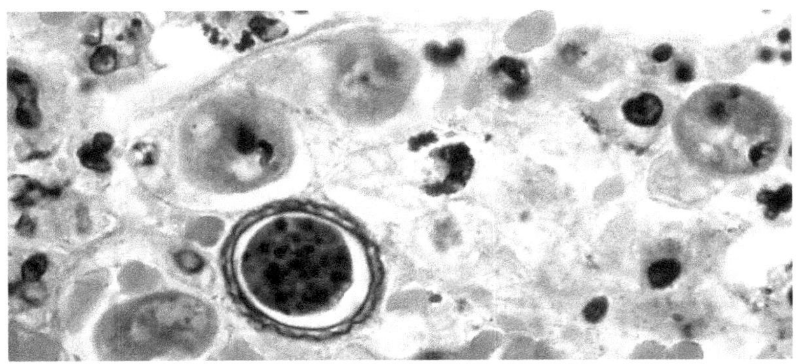

Acanthamoeba is a microscopic, free-living ameba, or amoeba* (single-celled living organism), that can cause rare**, but severe infections of the eye, skin, and central nervous system. The ameba is found worldwide in the environment in water and soil. The ameba can be spread to the eyes through contact lens use, cuts, or skin wounds or by being inhaled into the lungs. Most people will be exposed to Acanthamoeba during their lifetime, but very few will become sick from this exposure. The three diseases caused by Acanthamoeba are:

Acanthamoeba keratitis – An infection of the eye that typically occurs in healthy persons and can result in permanent visual impairment or blindness.

Granulomatous Amebic Encephalitis (GAE) – A serious infection of the brain and spinal cord that typically occurs in persons with a compromised immune system.

Disseminated infection – A widespread infection that can affect the skin, sinuses, lungs, and other organs independently or in combination. It is also more common in persons with a compromised immune system.

Image: This photomicrograph depicted a magnified view of brain tissue within which was a centrally located Acanthamoeba sp. cyst. Credit: DPDx

African Trypanosomiasis

African Trypanosomiasis, also known as "sleeping sickness," is caused by microscopic parasites of the species Trypanosoma brucei. It is transmitted by the tsetse fly (Glossina species), which is found only in rural Africa. Although the infection is not found in the United States, historically, it has been a serious public health problem in some regions of sub-Saharan Africa. Currently, about 10,000 new cases each year are reported to the World Health organization; however, it is believed that many cases go undiagnosed and unreported. Sleeping sickness is curable with medication but is fatal if left untreated.

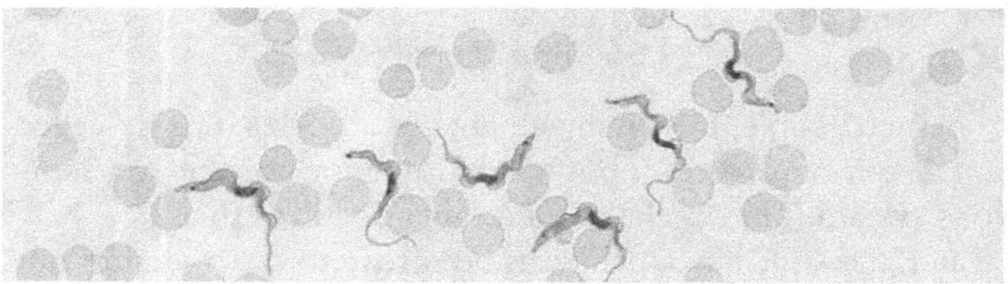

Image: Trypanosoma brucei rhodesiense in a Giemsa-stained blood smear. (Credit: DPDx)

Echinococcosis

Echinococcosis is a parasitic disease caused by infection with tiny tapeworms of the genus Echinococcus. Echinococcosis is classified as either cystic echinococcosis or alveolar echinococcosis.

Cystic echinocccosis (CE), also known as hydatid disease, is caused by infection with the larval stage of Echinococcus granulosus, a ~2-7-millimeter-long tapeworm found in dogs (definitive host) and sheep, cattle, goats, and pigs (intermediate hosts). Although most infections in humans are asymptomatic, CE causes harmful, slowly enlarging cysts in the liver, lungs, and other organs that often grow unnoticed and neglected for years.

Alveolar echinococcosis (AE) disease is caused by infection with the larval stage of Echinococcus multilocularis, a ~1-4-millimeter-long tapeworm found in foxes, coyotes, and dogs (definitive hosts). Small rodents are intermediate hosts for E. multilocularis. Although cases of AE in animals in endemic areas are relatively common, human cases are rare. AE poses a much greater health threat to people than CE, causing parasitic tumors that can form in the liver, lungs, brain, and other organs. If left untreated, AE can be fatal.

Image: L to R: Echinococcus granulosus adult, stained with carmine. Close-up of the scolex of E. granulosus. In this focal plane, one of the suckers is clearly visible, as is the ring of rostellar hooks. Credit: DPDx

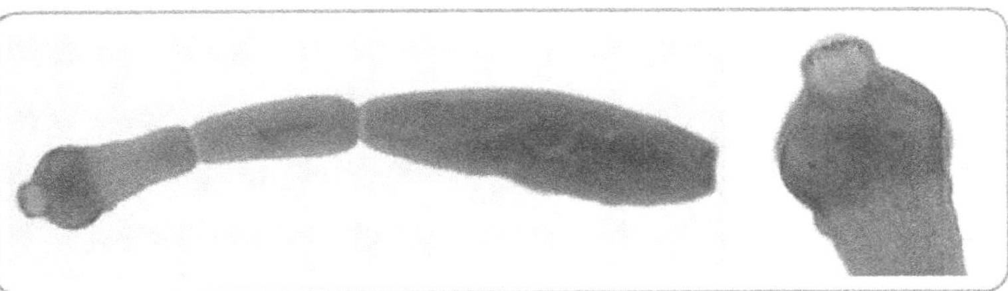

Echinococcosis

Amebiasis - Entamoeba histolytica Infection

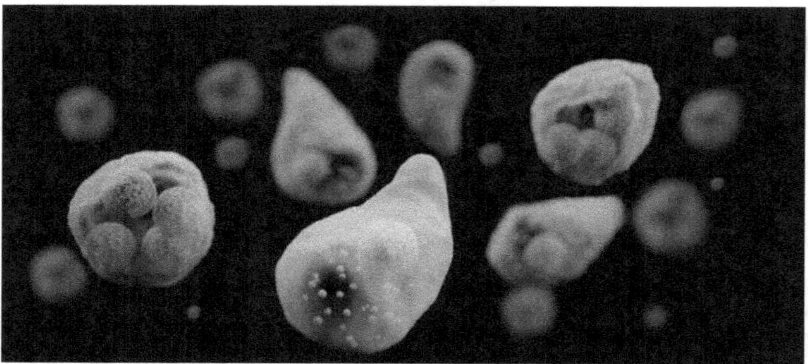

Amebiasis is a disease caused by the parasite Entamoeba histolytica. It can affect anyone, although it is more common in people who live in tropical areas with poor sanitary conditions. Diagnosis can be difficult because other parasites can look very similar to E. histolytica when seen under a microscope. Infected people do not always become sick. If your doctor determines that you are infected and need treatment, medication is available.

American Trypanosomiasis (also known as Chagas Disease)

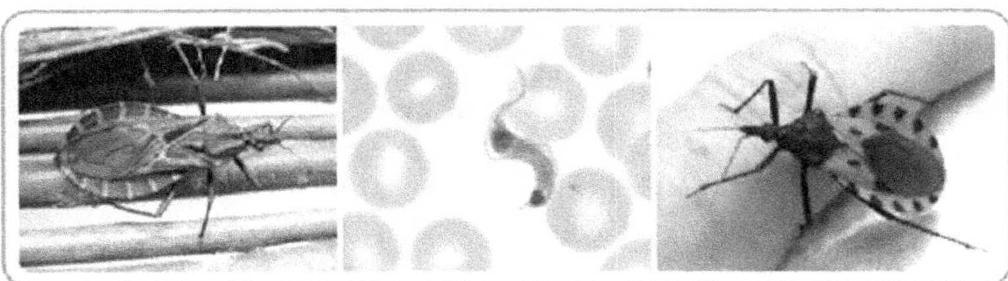

Above Images: Left and Right: Various species of triatomine bugs, which if infected can transmit T. cruzi. Center: T. cruzi trypomastigote in a thin blood smear stained with Giemsa. Credit: DPDx

Chagas disease is named after the Brazilian physician Carlos Chagas, who discovered the disease in 1909. It is caused by the parasite Trypanosoma cruzi, which is transmitted to animals and people by insect vectors and is found only in the Americas (mainly, in rural areas of Latin America where poverty is widespread). Chagas disease (T. cruzi infection) is also referred to as American trypanosomiasis.

Zoonotic Hookworm

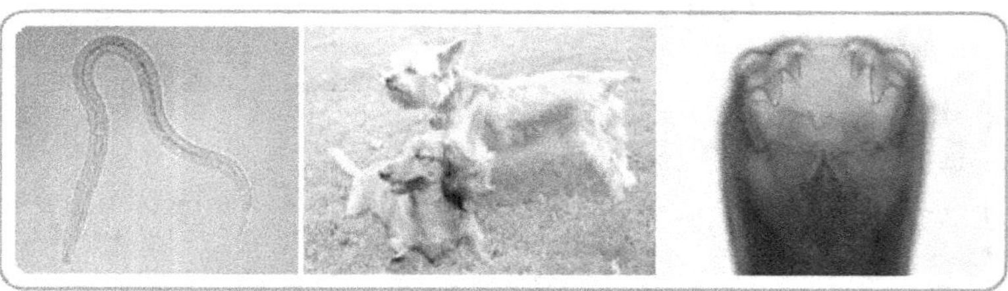

Zoonotic hookworms are hookworms that live in animals but can be transmitted to humans. Dogs and cats can become infected with several hookworm species, including Ancylostoma brazilense, A. caninum, A. ceylanicum, and Uncinaria stenocephala. The eggs of these parasites are shed in the feces of infected animals and can end up in the environment, contaminating the ground where the animal defecated. People become infected when the zoonotic hookworm larvae penetrate unprotected skin, especially when walking barefoot or sitting on contaminated soil or sand. This can result in a disease called cutaneous larva migrans (CLM), when the larvae migrate through the skin and cause inflammation.

Image: L: Filariform (L3) hookworm larvae. These L3 are found in the environment and infect the human host by penetration of the skin. Center: Two dogs playing. Worming your pet regularly will prevent zoonotic hookworm infection. R: Extreme magnification of the anterior end of an adult of Ancylostoma caninum, a dog parasite that has been found to produce a rare human infection known as eosinophilic enteritis. Credit: DPDx

Angiostrongyliasis (also known as Angiostrongylus Infection)

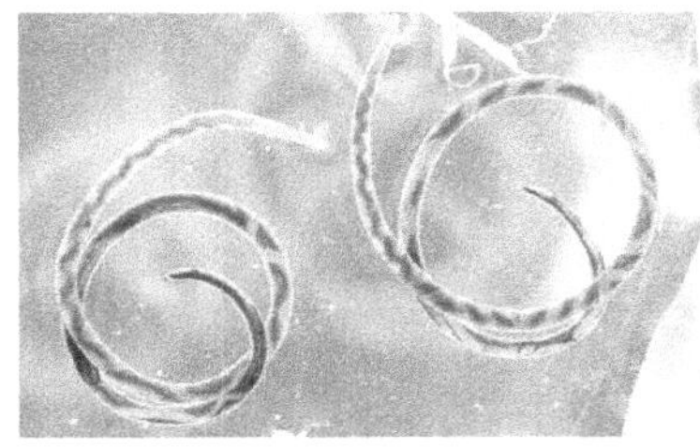 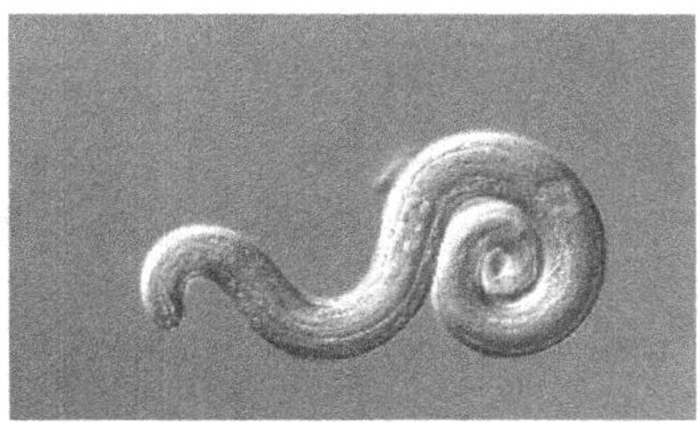

Images: Left: Two Angiostrongylus adult females recovered from rat lungs. The distinctive, coiled pattern seen in both worms is created by the white uterine tubes and red, blood-filled intestine. Right: Angiostrongylus cantonensis third-stage (L3), infective larva recovered from a slug. Image captured under differential interference contrast (DIC) microscopy. (Credit: DPDx)

Angiostrongylus is a parasitic nematode that can cause severe gastrointestinal or central nervous system disease in humans, depending on the species. Angiostrongylus cantonensis, which is also known as the rat lungworm, causes eosinophilic meningitis and is prevalent in Southeast Asia and tropical Pacific islands. The recognized distribution of the parasite has been increasing over time and infections have been identified in other areas, including Africa, the Caribbean, and the United States.

Anisakiasis

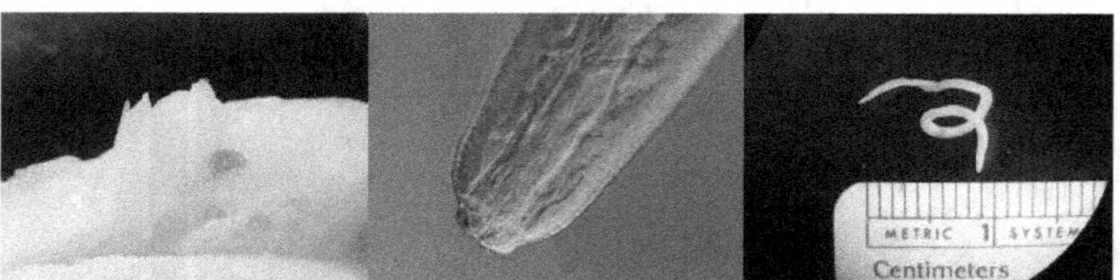

Images: Left: A coiled anisakid worm (Pseudoterranova decipiens) in a fillet of cod. Center: A view of the anterior (head) end of Pseudoterranova decipiens, showing the presence of "lips"; taken under differential interference contrast (DIC) microscopy. Right: Pseudoterranova decipiens recovered from a human patient. (Credit: DPDx)

Anisakiasis is a parasitic disease caused by anisakid nematodes (worms) that can invade the stomach wall or intestine of humans. The transmission of this disease occurs when infective larvae are ingested from fish or squid that humans eat raw or undercooked. In some cases, this infection is treated by removal of the larvae via endoscopy or surgery.

Ascariasis

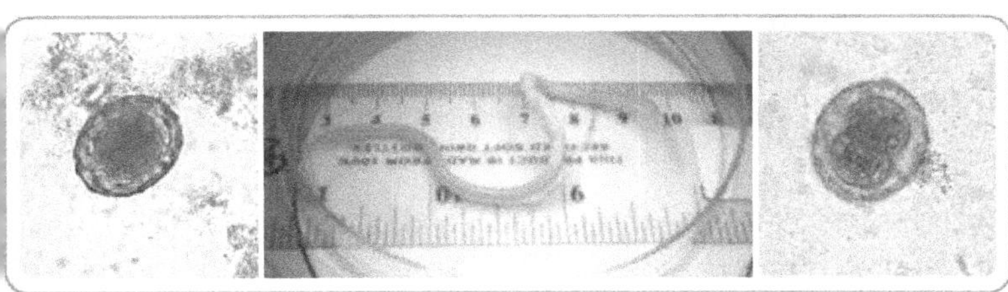

Image: Left/Right: Fertilized eggs of A. lumbricoides in unstained wet mounts of stool. Center: Adult female A. lumbricoides. Credit: DPDx, Orange County Public Health Laboratory, Santa Ana, CA.

An estimated 807 million–1.2 billion people in the world are infected with Ascaris lumbricoides (sometimes called just Ascaris or ascariasis). Ascaris, hookworm, and whipworm are parasitic worms known as soil-transmitted helminths (STH). Together, they account for a major burden of parasitic disease worldwide. Ascariasis is now uncommon in the United States. Ascaris parasites live in the intestine and Ascaris eggs are passed in the feces (poop) of infected people. If an infected person defecates outside (for example, near bushes, in a garden, or in a field), or if the feces of an infected person are used as fertilizer, eggs are deposited on soil. The eggs can then mature into a form of the parasite that is infective. Ascariasis is caused by ingesting eggs. This can happen when hands or fingers that have contaminated dirt on them are put in the mouth, or by consuming vegetables or fruits that have not been carefully cooked, washed, or peeled.

People infected with Ascaris often show no symptoms. If symptoms do occur, they can be light and include abdominal discomfort. Heavy infections can cause intestinal blockage and impair growth in children. Other symptoms such as cough are due to migration of the worms through the body. Ascariasis is treatable with medication prescribed by your health care provider.

Humans can also be infected by pig roundworm (Ascaris suum). Ascaris lumbricoides (human roundworm) and Ascaris suum (pig roundworm) are indistinguishable. It is unknown how many people worldwide are infected with Ascaris suum.

Babesiosis

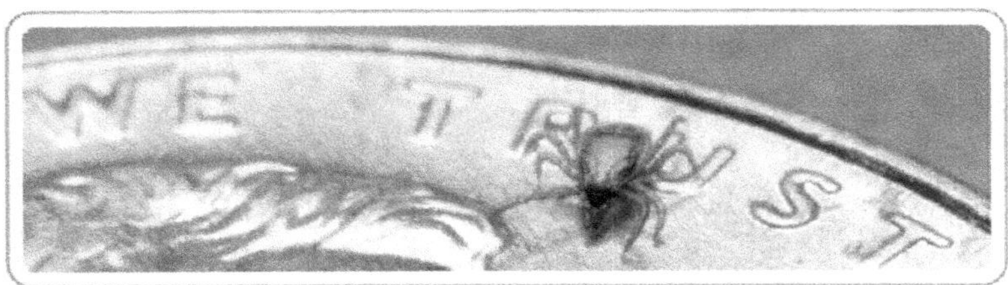

Babesia microti is transmitted by the bite of infected Ixodes scapularis ticks—typically, by the nymph stage of the tick, which is about the size of a poppy seed. An Ixodes scapularis nymph is shown on the face of a penny. (Credit: G. Hickling, University of Tennessee)

Babesiosis is caused by microscopic parasites that infect red blood cells and are spread by certain ticks. In the United States, tickborne transmission is most common in particular regions and seasons: it mainly occurs in parts of the Northeast and upper Midwest and usually peaks during the warm months. Although many people who are infected with Babesia do not have symptoms, for those who do effective treatment is available. Babesiosis is preventable, if simple steps are taken to reduce exposure to ticks.

Balantidiasis (also known as Balantidium coli Infection)

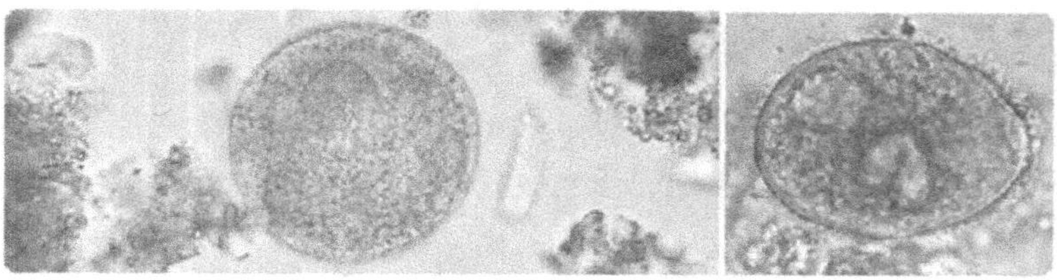

Images: Left: Balantidium coli cyst. Right: B. coli trophozoite in a wet mount of feces. (Credit: DPDx)

Balantidium coli, though rare in the US, is an intestinal protozoan parasite that can infect humans. These parasites can be transmitted through the fecal-oral route by contaminated food and water. Balantidium coli infection is mostly asymptomatic, but people with other serious illnesses can experience persistent diarrhea, abdominal pain, and sometimes a perforated colon. When traveling to endemic tropical countries, Balantidium coli infection can be prevented by following good hygiene practices. Wash all fruits and vegetables with clean water when preparing or eating them, even if they have a removable skin.

Balamuthia mandrillaris - Granulomatous Amebic Encephalitis (GAE)

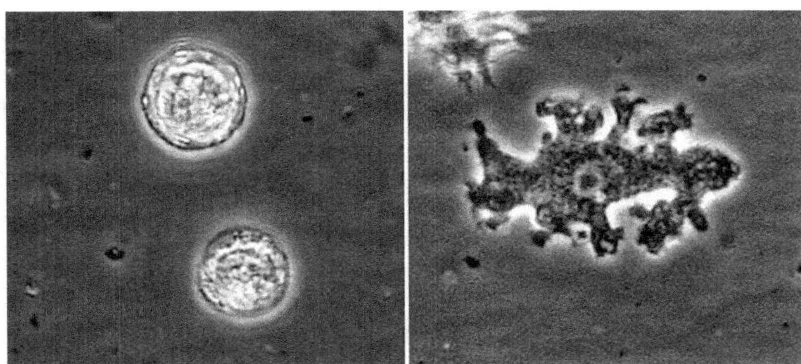

Balamuthia mandrillaris is a free-living ameba (a single-celled living organism) naturally found in the environment. Balamuthia can cause a rare* and serious infection of the brain and spinal cord called Granulomatous Amebic Encephalitis (GAE).

Baylisascaris infection

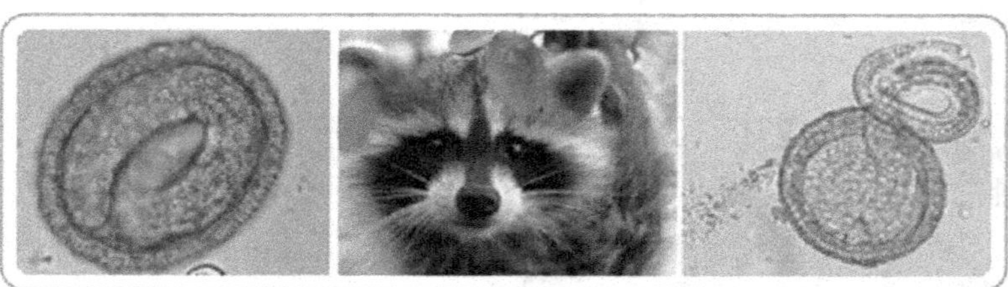

Image: Left: Embryonated B. procyonis egg, showing the developing larva inside. Right: Larva of B. procyonis hatching from an egg. Center: Raccoons are hosts for the roundworms that can cause Baylisascaris infection. Credit: DPDx, U.S. Fish & Wildlife ServiceExternal

Baylisascaris infection is caused by a roundworm found in raccoons. This roundworm can infect people as well as a variety of other animals, including dogs. Human infections are rare but can be severe if the parasites invade the eye (ocular larva migrans), organs (visceral larva migrans) or the brain (neural larva migrans).

Bed bugs,

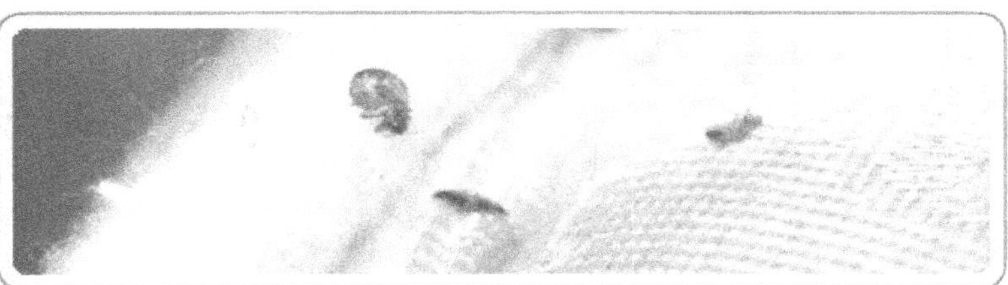

Image: Bed bugs hiding in the ribbing of a mattress corner.

Bed bugs, a problem worldwide, are resurging, causing property loss, expense, and inconvenience. The good news is that bed bugs do not transmit disease. The best way to prevent bed bugs is regular inspection for signs of an infestation.

Schistosomiasis

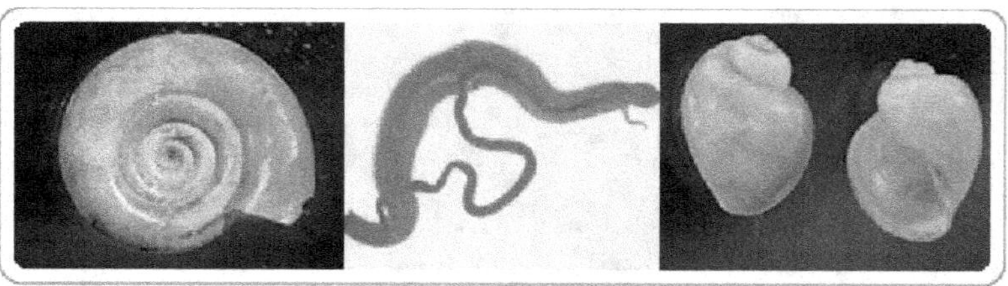

Image: Left: Biomphalaria sp., the intermediate host for S. mansoni. Right: Bulinus sp., the intermediate host for S. haematobium and S. intercalatum. Center: Adults of S. mansoni. The thin female resides in the gynecophoral canal of the thicker male. Credit: DPDx

Schistosomiasis, also known as bilharzia, is a disease caused by parasitic worms. Although the worms that cause schistosomiasis are not found in the United States, people are infected worldwide. In terms of impact this disease is second only to malaria as the most devastating parasitic disease. Schistosomiasis is considered one of the neglected tropical diseases (NTDs).

The parasites that cause schistosomiasis live in certain types of freshwater snails. The infectious form of the parasite, known as cercariae, emerge from the snail into the water. You can become infected when your skin encounters contaminated freshwater. Most human infections are caused by Schistosoma mansoni, S. haematobium, or S. japonicum.

Blastocystis spp. Infection

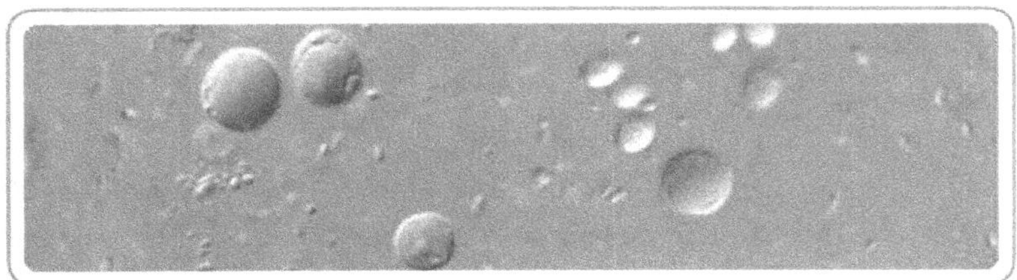

Image: B. spp. cyst-like forms in wet mounts under differential interference contrast (DIC) microscopy. Credit: DPDx

Blastocystis is a common microscopic organism that inhabits the intestine and is found throughout the world. A full understanding of the biology of Blastocystis and its relationship to other organisms is not clear but is an active area of research.

Blastocystis spp. FAQs

What is Blastocystis spp.?
Blastocystis is a common microscopic organism that inhabits the intestine and is found throughout the world. A full understanding of the biology of Blastocystis and its relationship to other organisms is not clear but is an active area of research. Infection with Blastocystis is called blastocystosis.

What are the symptoms of infection with Blastocystis?
Watery or loose stools, diarrhea, abdominal pain, anal itching, weight loss, constipation, and excess gas have all been reported in persons with Blastocystis infection. Many people have no symptoms at all. The organism can be found in both well and sick persons.

How long will I be infected?
Blastocystis can remain in the intestine for weeks, months, or years

Is Blastocystis spp. the cause of my symptoms?
The role of Blastocystis in causing disease is controversial among experts. Some types of Blastocystis may be more likely to be associated with symptoms. Finding Blastocystis in stool samples should be followed up with a careful search for other possible causes of your symptoms.

Is having blastocystosis common?
Yes. In fact, many people have Blastocystis in their intestine, some without ever having symptoms.

What should I do if I think I have blastocystosis?
See your health care provider who will ask you to provide stool samples for testing. Diagnosis may be difficult, so you may be asked to submit several stool samples.

Is medication available to treat blastocystosis?
Yes. Drugs are available by prescription to treat blastocystosis. However, sometimes medication is not effective, and a search for other possible causes of your symptoms may be necessary.

How did I get blastocystosis?

How Blastocystis is transmitted is not known for certain, although the number of people infected seems to increase in areas where sanitation and personal hygiene is not adequate. Studies have suggested that risk of infection may increase through:

ingesting contaminated food or water,
exposure to a day care environment, or
exposure to animals.

How can I prevent infection with Blastocystis?
Wash your hands with soap and warm water after using the toilet, changing diapers, and before handling food.
Teach children the importance of washing hands to prevent infection.

Avoid water or food that may be contaminated.
Wash and peel all raw vegetables and fruits before eating.
When traveling in countries where the water supply may be unsafe, avoid drinking unboiled tap water and avoid uncooked foods washed with unboiled tap water. Bottled or canned carbonated beverages, seltzers, pasteurized fruit drinks, and steaming hot coffee and tea are safe to drink.
More on: Handwashing

Should I be concerned about spreading infection to the rest of my household?

There is little risk of spreading infection if you practice adequate personal hygiene. This includes thorough hand washing with soap and warm water after using the toilet and before handling food.

Biology
Causal Agents

Blastocystis is a genetically diverse unicellular parasite of unclear pathogenic potential that colonizes the intestines of humans and a wide range of non-human animals. Based on molecular data, the organism has been classified as a stramenopile. Organisms such as diatoms, chrysophytes, water molds, and slime nets are other examples of stramenopiles.

Blastocystis organisms isolated from humans have commonly been referred to as B. hominis. However, because of extensive genetic diversity (even among organisms isolated from humans) and low host specificity, the designation Blastocystis sp. is considered more appropriate. If genetic typing is performed, the subtype (ST) also should be noted in accordance with consensus terminology.* Among the nine STs found to date in humans, the four most prevalent STs are ST1, ST2, ST3, and ST4; other STs occur sporadically and may be related to zoonotic transmission.

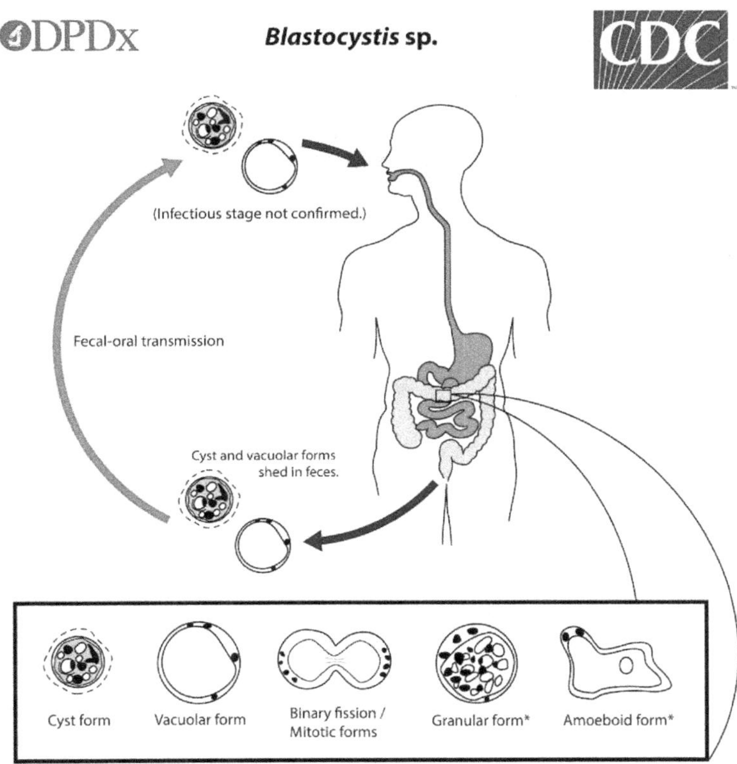

*Various forms that may occasionally be seen in human stool samples and in culture.
Their biological significance is not well understood.

The life cycle of Blastocystis sp. is not yet understood, including the infectious stage and whether (and which of the) various morphologic forms of this polymorphic organism that have been identified in stool or culture constitute distinct biologic stages of the parasite in the intestinal tract of hosts. The cyst form (3–5 µm) is postulated to be an infectious stage, but not confirmed. The predominant form found in human stool specimens is referred to as the vacuolar (or central body) form and is of variable size (5–40 µm, occasionally much larger). Replication appears to occur via binary fission. Other morphologic forms (e.g., ameboid and granular forms) also have been noted in stool samples and/or culture; their biological role and eventual developmental fate require further investigation.

Body lice

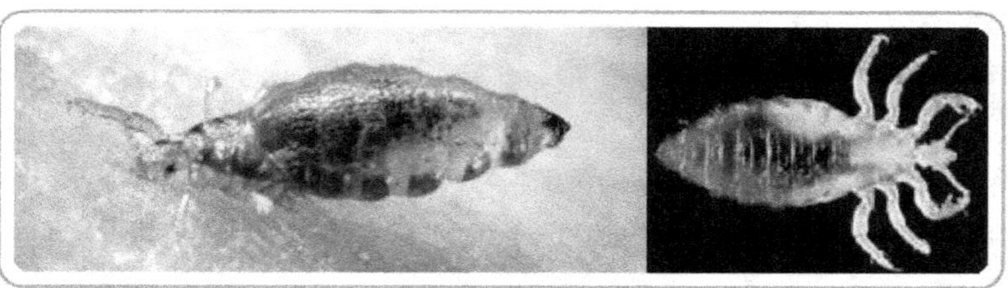

Image: Pictures of two adult body lice. Credit: PHIL, CDC

Adult body lice are 2.3–3.6 mm in length. Body lice live and lay eggs on clothing and only move to the skin to feed.
Body lice are known to spread disease.

Body lice infestations (pediculosis) are spread most commonly by close person-to-person contact but are generally limited to persons who live under conditions of crowding and poor hygiene (for example, the homeless, refugees, etc.). Dogs, cats, and other pets do not play a role in the transmission of human lice.

Improved hygiene and access to regular changes of clean clothes is the only treatment needed for body lice infestations.

Capillariasis (also known as Capillaria Infection)

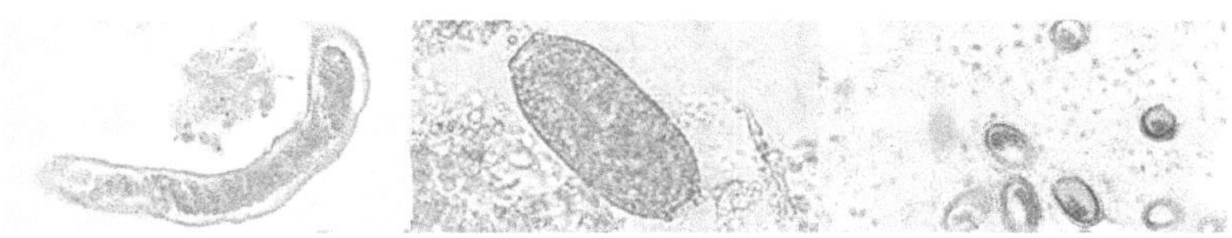

Images: Left: Longitudinal section of an adult of C. philippinensis from an intestinal biopsy specimen stained with hematoxylin and eosin (H&E) Middle: Egg of C. philippinensis in stool. Right: A cross-section through eggs of C. hepatica in liver tissue. (Credit: DPDx)

Capillariasis is a parasitic disease in humans caused by two different species of capillarids: Capillaria hepatica and Capillaria philippinensis. C. hepatica is transferred through the fecal matter of infected animals and can lead to hepatitis. C. philippinensis is transferred through ingesting infected small freshwater fish and can lead to diarrhea and emaciation.

Cercarial Dermatitis (also known as Swimmer's Itch)

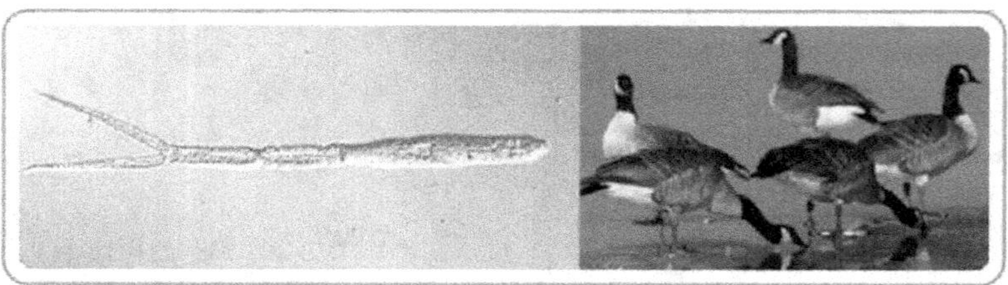

Swimmer's itch, also called cercarial dermatitis, appears as a skin rash caused by an allergic reaction to certain parasites that infect some birds and mammals. These microscopic parasites are released from infected snails into fresh and saltwater (such as lakes, ponds, and oceans). While the parasite's preferred host is the specific bird or mammal, if the parasite encounters a swimmer, it burrows into the skin causing an allergic reaction and rash. Swimmer's itch is found throughout the world and is more frequent during summer months. Most cases of swimmer's itch do not require medical attention. Image: Left: Cercariae of Austrobilharzia variglandis (left), which can cause cercarial dermatitis. Note the forked "tail" and a pair of "eye spots" near the anterior end (right). Right: A group of geese, a preferred host of the parasite that causes cercarial dermatitis. Credit: DPDx

American Trypanosomiasis (also known as Chagas Disease)

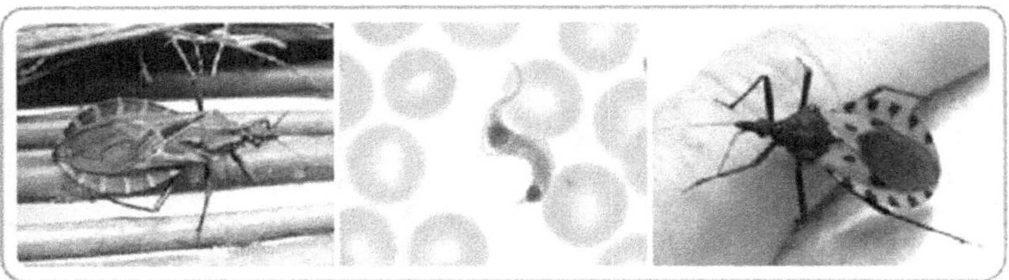

Above Images: Left and Right: Various species of triatomine bugs, which if infected can transmit T. cruzi. Center: T. cruzi trypomastigote in a thin blood smear stained with Giemsa. Credit: DPDx

Chagas disease is named after the Brazilian physician Carlos Chagas, who discovered the disease in 1909. It is caused by the parasite Trypanosoma cruzi, which is transmitted to animals and people by insect vectors and is found only in the Americas (mainly, in rural areas of Latin America where poverty is widespread). Chagas disease (T. cruzi infection) is also referred to as American trypanosomiasis.

Nonpathogenic (Harmless) Intestinal Protozoa

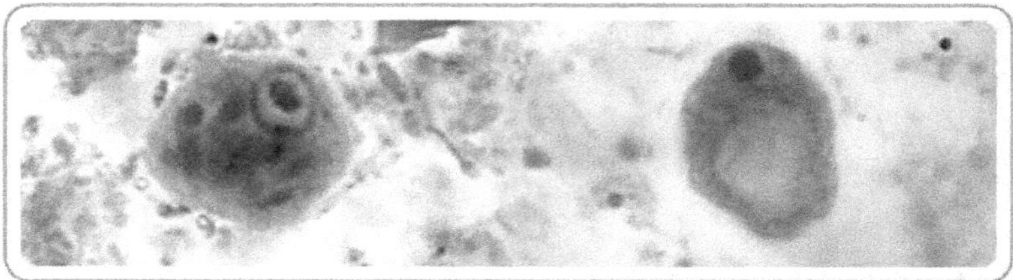

Image: Left: Entamoeba polecki cyst stained with trichrome. Right: Iodamoeba buetschlii cyst stained with trichrome. (Credit: DPDx)

Nonpathogenic intestinal protozoa are single-celled parasites commonly found in the intestinal tract but never associated with illness. They do not harm the body, even in people with weak immune systems. Symptomatic people who are found to have these protozoa in their stool should be examined for other causes of their symptoms.

The nonpathogenic intestinal protozoa include:

Chilomastix mesnili
Endolimax nana
Entamoeba coli
Entamoeba dispar
Entamoeba hartmanni
Entamoeba polecki
Iodamoeba buetschlii

Clonorchis

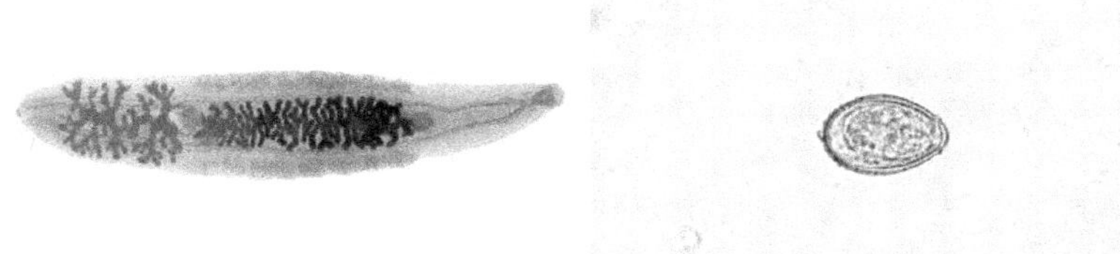

Images: Left: Adult of C. sinensis, stained with carmine. Right: C. sinensis egg in a fecal sample. (Credit: DPDx)

Clonorchis is a liver fluke parasite that humans can get by eating raw or undercooked fish, crabs, or crayfish from areas where the parasite is found. Found across parts of Asia, Clonorchis is also known as the Chinese or oriental liver fluke. Liver flukes infect the liver, gallbladder, and bile duct in humans. While most infected persons do not show any symptoms, infections that last a long time can result in severe symptoms and serious illness. Untreated, infections may persist for up to 25–30 years, the lifespan of the parasite.

Diagnosis of Clonorchis infection is based on microscopic identification of the parasite's eggs in stool specimens. Safe and effective medication is available to treat Clonorchis infections. Adequately freezing or cooking fish will kill the parasite.

Zoonotic Hookworm

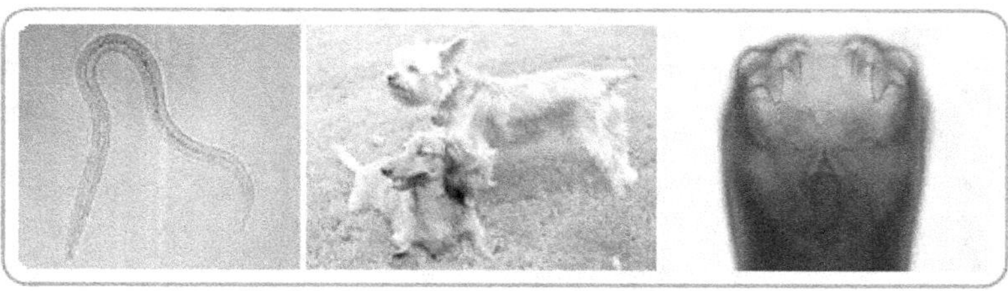

Zoonotic hookworms are hookworms that live in animals but can be transmitted to humans. Dogs and cats can become infected with several hookworm species, including Ancylostoma brazilense, A. caninum, A. ceylanicum, and Uncinaria stenocephala. The eggs of these parasites are shed in the feces of infected animals and can end up in the environment, contaminating the ground where the animal defecated. People become infected when the zoonotic hookworm larvae penetrate unprotected skin, especially when walking barefoot or sitting on contaminated soil or sand. This can result in a disease called cutaneous larva migrans (CLM), when the larvae migrate through the skin and cause inflammation.

Image: L: Filariform (L3) hookworm larvae. These L3 are found in the environment and infect the human host by penetration of the skin. Center: Two dogs playing. Worming your pet regularly will prevent zoonotic hookworm infection. R: Extreme magnification of the anterior end of an adult of Ancylostoma caninum, a dog parasite that has been found to produce a rare human infection known as eosinophilic enteritis. Credit: DPDx

Pubic "Crab" Lice

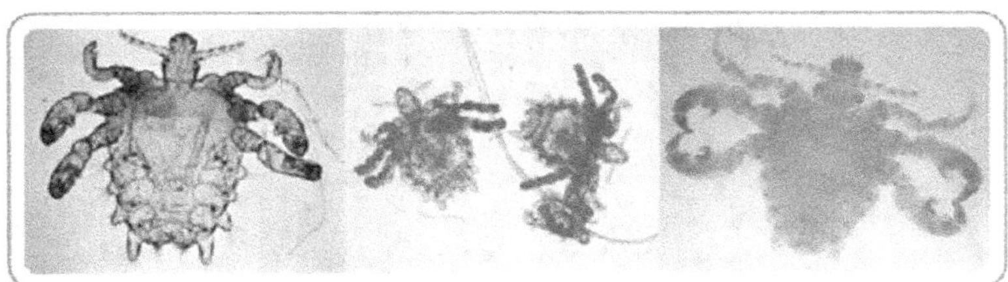

Adult pubic lice are 1.1–1.8 mm in length. Pubic lice typically are found attached to hair in the pubic area but sometimes are found on coarse hair elsewhere on the body (for example, eyebrows, eyelashes, beard, mustache, chest, armpits, etc.).

Pubic lice infestations (pthiriasis) are usually spread through sexual contact. Dogs, cats, and other pets do not play a role in the transmission of human pubic lice.

Both over-the-counter and prescription medications are available for treatment of pubic lice infestations.

Image: Pictures of pubic "crab" lice. The vernacular name comes from their crab like claws and body shape. Credit: PHIL, DPDx.

Cryptosporidium (also known as "Crypto")

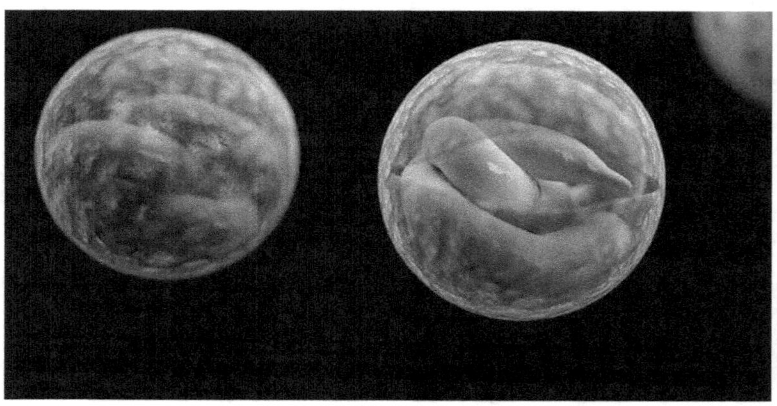

Cryptosporidium is a microscopic parasite that causes the diarrheal disease cryptosporidiosis. Both the parasite and the disease are commonly known as "Crypto."

There are many species of Cryptosporidium that infect animals, some of which also infect humans. The parasite is protected by an outer shell that allows it to survive outside the body for long periods of time and makes it very tolerant to chlorine disinfection.

While this parasite can be spread in several different ways, water (drinking water and recreational water) is the most common way to spread the parasite. Cryptosporidium is a leading cause of waterborne disease among humans in the United States.

Cyclosporiasis (Cyclospora Infection)

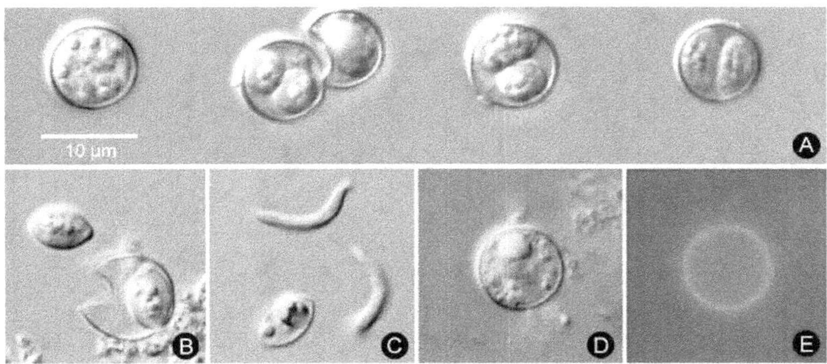

Images: Infected people shed unsporulated (non-infective; immature) Cyclospora cayetanensis oocysts in their stool; immature oocysts usually require at least 1–2 weeks under favorable laboratory conditions to sporulate and become infective. An unsporulated oocyst, with undifferentiated cytoplasm, is shown (far left), next to a sporulating oocyst that contains two immature sporocysts (A). An oocyst that was mechanically ruptured has released one of its two sporocysts (B). One free sporocyst is shown as well as two free sporozoites, the infective stage of the parasite (C). Oocysts (D) are auto-fluorescent when viewed under ultraviolet microscopy (E). (Credit: CDC/DPDx)

Cyclosporiasis is an intestinal illness caused by the microscopic parasite Cyclospora cayetanensis. People can become infected with Cyclospora by consuming food or water contaminated with the parasite. People living or traveling in countries where cyclosporiasis is endemic may be at increased risk for infection.

Cysticercosis

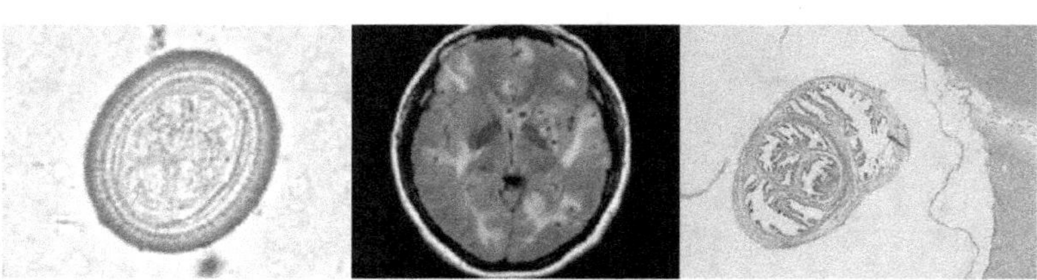

Images: Left: Taenia egg at a high magnification of 400x. When consumed by humans, Taenia solium eggs can lead to cysticercosis, including a serious condition known as neurocysticercosis. Center: A radiographic image of the brain of a patient who has neurocysticercosis; the small dark spots within the brain are larval cysts of T. solium. Right: A cross-section through a T. solium cyst from a human brain tissue specimen, stained with hematoxylin and eosin (H&E). (Credit (L to R): Westchester Medical Center, PHIL, DPDx.)

Cysticercosis is a parasitic tissue infection caused by larval cysts of the tapeworm Taenia solium. These larval cysts infect brain, muscle, or other tissue, and are a major cause of adult onset seizures in most low-income countries. A person gets cysticercosis by swallowing eggs found in the feces of a person who has an intestinal tapeworm. People living in the same household with someone who has a tapeworm have a much higher risk of getting cysticercosis than people who don't. People do not get cysticercosis by eating undercooked pork. Eating undercooked pork can result in intestinal tapeworm if the pork contains larval cysts. Pigs become infected by eating tapeworm eggs in the feces of a human infected with a tapeworm. Both the tapeworm infection, also known as taeniasis, and cysticercosis occur globally. The highest rates of infection are found in areas of Latin America, Asia, and Africa that have poor sanitation and free-ranging pigs that have access to human feces. Although uncommon, cysticercosis can occur in people who have never traveled outside of the United States. For example, a person infected with a tapeworm who does not wash his or her hands might accidentally contaminate food with tapeworm eggs while preparing it for others.

In the United States, cysticercosis is considered one of the Neglected Parasitic Infections (NPIs), a group of five parasitic diseases that have been targeted by CDC for public health action.

Cystoisosporiasis (formerly known as Isosporiasis)

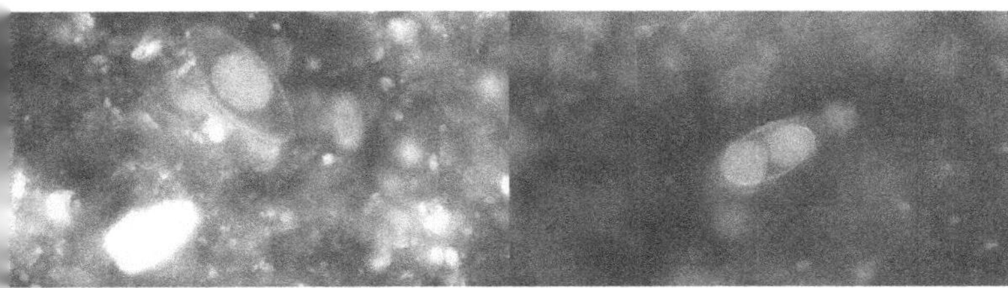

Images: Two immature oocysts of Cystoisospora belli in unstained wet mounts viewed by ultraviolet (UV) fluorescence microscopy. The oocyst on the left contains one sporoblast; the oocyst on the right contains two sporoblasts. (Credit: DPDx)

Cystoisosporiasis (formerly known as isosporiasis) is an intestinal disease of humans caused by the coccidian parasite Cystoisospora belli (formerly known as Isospora belli). Cystoisosporiasis is most common in tropical and subtropical areas of the world. The parasite can be spread by ingesting contaminated food or water. The most common symptom is watery diarrhea. The infection is treatable and preventable.

Dientamoeba fragilis

Dientamoeba fragilis is a parasite that lives in the large intestine of people. This protozoan parasite produces trophozoites; cysts have not been identified. The intestinal infection may be either asymptomatic or symptomatic.
Image: Binucleate (left) and uninucleate (right) trophozoites of D. fragilis, stained with trichrome. (Credit: DPDx).

Diphyllobothrium Infection

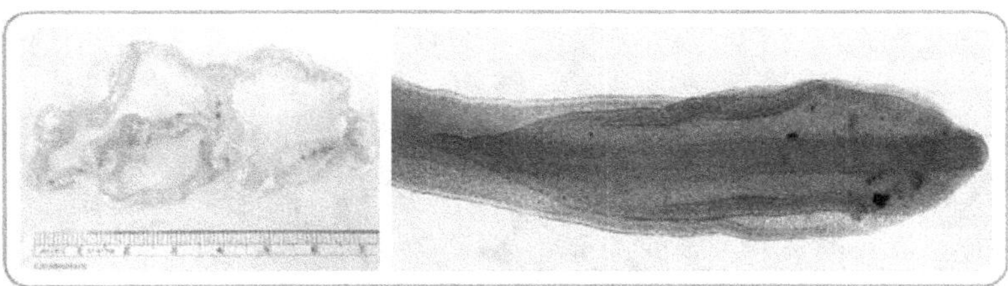

Diphyllobothrium latum and related species (the fish or broad tapeworm), the largest tapeworms that can infect people, can grow up to 30 feet long. While most infections are asymptomatic, complications include intestinal obstruction and gall bladder disease caused by migration of proglottids. Diagnosis is made by identification of eggs or segments of the tapeworm in a stool sample with a microscope. Safe and effective medications are available to treat Diphyllobothrium. Infections are acquired by eating raw or undercooked fish, usually from the Northern Hemisphere (Europe, newly independent states of the Former Soviet Union, North America, Asia), but cases have also been reported in Uganda and Chile. Fish infected with Diphyllobothrium larvae may be transported to and consumed in any area of the world. Adequately freezing or cooking fish will kill the parasite.

Image: L: Section of an adult D. latum containing many proglottids. The scolex was not present in this specimen. Scale is in centimeters. R: Scolex of D. latum. Credit: Florida State Public Health Laboratory, DPDx

Dipylidium Infection (also known as Dog and Cat Flea Tapeworm)

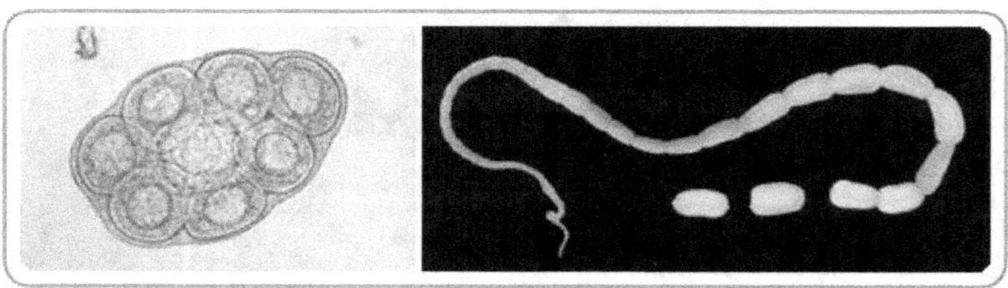

Dipylidium is tapeworm of cats and dogs. People become infected when they accidentally swallow a flea infected with tapeworm larvae; most reported cases involve children. Dipylidium infection is easily treated in humans and animals.

Image: Left: D. caninum egg packet, containing 8 visible eggs, in a wet mount. Right: Adult tapeworm of D. caninum. The scolex of the worm is very narrow and the proglottids, as they mature, get larger. Credit: DPDx

Dirofilaria immitis

Images: Left: A cross-section through a Dirofilaria immitis adult female in a human tissue biopsy specimen, stained with hematoxylin and eosin. Right: A cross-section through a coiled adult female Dirofilaria tenuis, also in a human tissue biopsy. (Credit: DPDx)

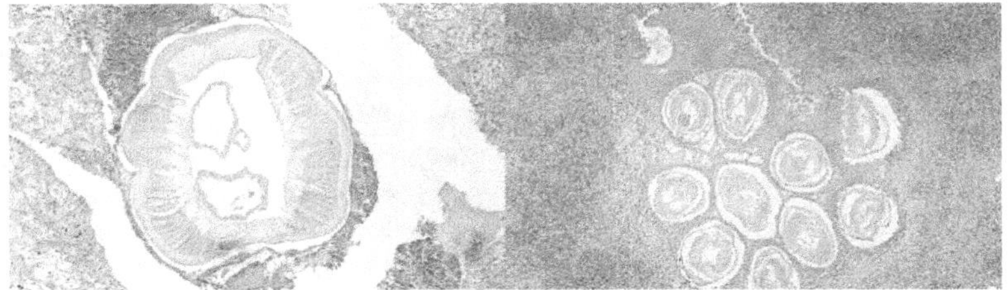

Latest on Guinea Worm Eradication:

The program has made great strides from 3.5 million cases annually in the mid-1980s to 28 human cases in 2018. Global eradication is within reach.

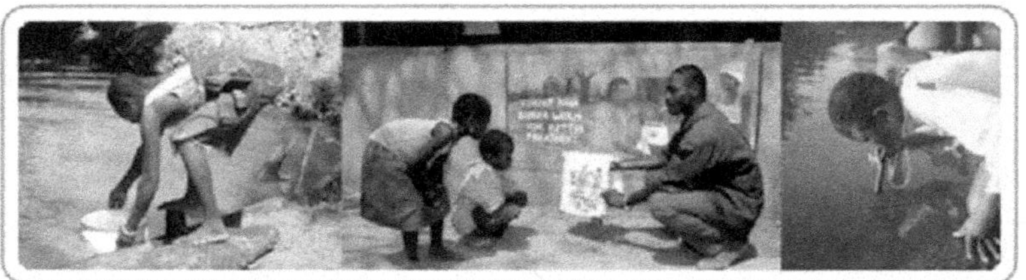

Guinea worm disease, a Neglected Tropical Disease (NTD), is caused by the parasite Dracunculus medinensis. The disease affects poor communities in remote parts of Africa that do not have safe water to drink. There is neither a drug treatment for Guinea worm disease nor a vaccine to prevent it. Great progress has been made towards elimination of Guinea worm disease; the number of human cases annually has fallen from 3.5 million in the mid-1980s to 28 in 2018.

Above Images: Left: Woman gathering water in a pond. Guinea worm disease is transmitted by drinking unfiltered water from ponds and other stagnant surface water sources. Center: A health worker providing education to children about how to avoid getting Guinea worm disease. Right: A young man using a pipe filter to drink from a pond. Pipe filters help remove the water fleas that carry Dracunculus medinensis. Credit: CDC PHIL, The Carter Centerexternal icon

Echinococcosis

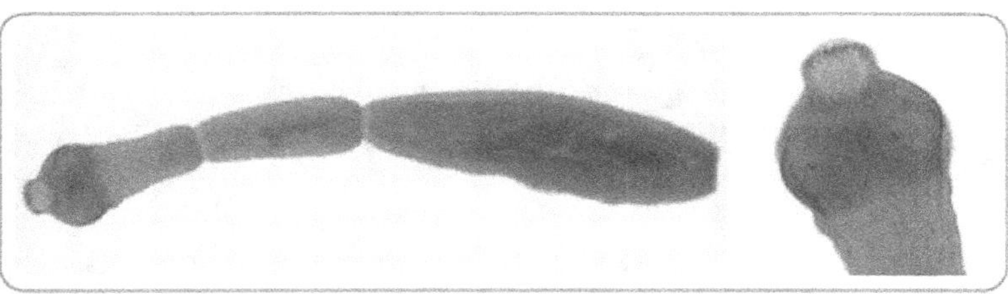

Echinococcosis is a parasitic disease caused by infection with tiny tapeworms of the genus Echinococcus. Echinococcosis is classified as either cystic echinococcosis or alveolar echinococcosis.

Cystic echinocccosis (CE), also known as hydatid disease, is caused by infection with the larval stage of Echinococcus granulosus, a ~2-7-millimeter-long tapeworm found in dogs (definitive host) and sheep, cattle, goats, and pigs (intermediate hosts). Although most infections in humans are asymptomatic, CE causes harmful, slowly enlarging cysts in the liver, lungs, and other organs that often grow unnoticed and neglected for years.

Alveolar echinococcosis (AE) disease is caused by infection with the larval stage of Echinococcus multilocularis, a ~1-4-millimeter-long tapeworm found in foxes, coyotes, and dogs (definitive hosts). Small rodents are intermediate hosts for E. multilocularis. Although cases of AE in animals in endemic areas are relatively common, human cases are rare. AE poses a much greater health threat to people than CE, causing parasitic tumors that can form in the liver, lungs, brain, and other organs. If left untreated, AE can be fatal.

Image: L to R: Echinococcus granulosus adult, stained with carmine. Close-up of the scolex of E. granulosus. In this focal plane, one of the suckers is clearly visible, as is the ring of rostellar hooks. Credit: DPDx

Lymphatic Filariasis

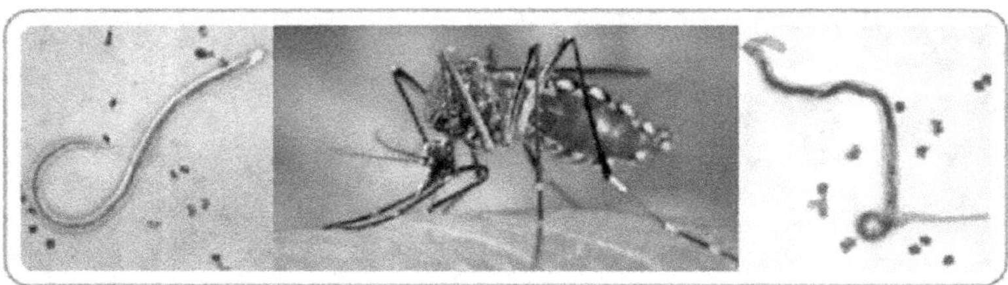

Lymphatic filariasis, considered globally as a neglected tropical disease (NTD), is a parasitic disease caused by microscopic, thread-like worms. The adult worms only live in the human lymph system. The lymph system maintains the body's fluid balance and fights infections. Lymphatic filariasis is spread from person to person by mosquitoes.

People with the disease can suffer from lymphedema and elephantiasis and in men, swelling of the scrotum, called hydrocele. Lymphatic filariasis is a leading cause of permanent disability worldwide. Communities frequently shun and reject women and men disfigured by the disease. Affected people frequently are unable to work because of their disability, and this harms their families and their communities.

Image: Left: Microfilaria of Wuchereria bancrofti in thick blood smear stained with Giemsa. Right: Microfilaria of Brugia malayi in a thick blood smear, stained with Giemsa. Center: Photograph of a female Aedes aegypti mosquito as she was in the process of obtaining a "blood meal." Laboratory strains of Aedes aegypti can be infected with Brugia. Credit: DPDx, PHIL

Nonpathogenic (Harmless) Intestinal Protozoa

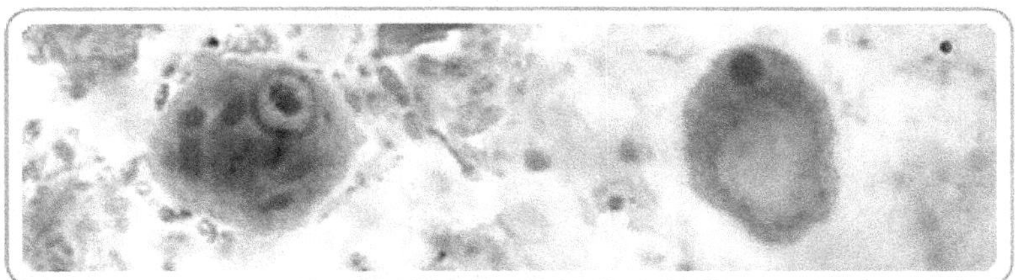

Nonpathogenic intestinal protozoa are single-celled parasites commonly found in the intestinal tract but never associated with illness. They do not harm the body, even in people with weak immune systems. Symptomatic people who are found to have these protozoa in their stool should be examined for other causes of their symptoms.

The nonpathogenic intestinal protozoa include:

Chilomastix mesnili
Endolimax nana
Entamoeba coli
Entamoeba dispar
Entamoeba hartmanni
Entamoeba polecki
Iodamoeba buetschlii

Image: Left: Entamoeba polecki cyst stained with trichrome. Right: Iodamoeba buetschlii cyst stained with trichrome. (Credit: DPDx)

Amebiasis - Entamoeba histolytica Infection

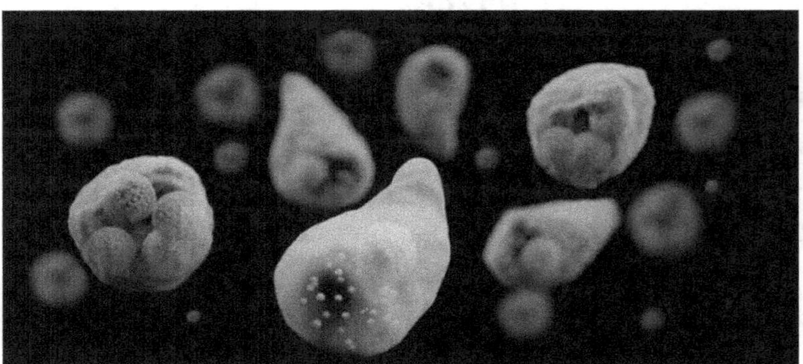

Amebiasis is a disease caused by the parasite Entamoeba histolytica. It can affect anyone, although it is more common in people who live in tropical areas with poor sanitary conditions. Diagnosis can be difficult because other parasites can look very similar to E. histolytica when seen under a microscope. Infected people do not always become sick. If your doctor determines that you are infected and need treatment, medication is available.

Enterobiasis (also known as Pinworm Infection)

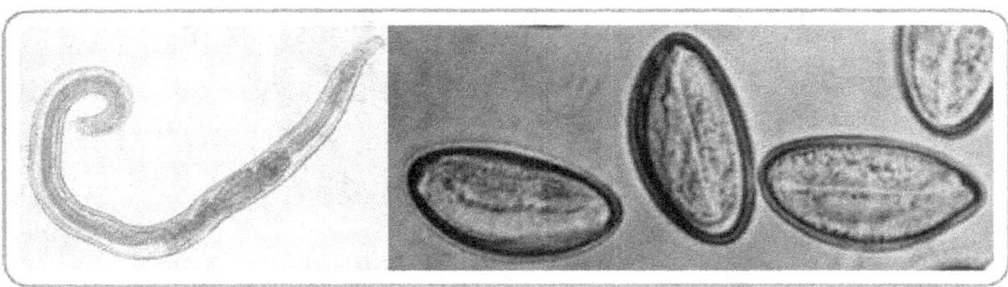

Pinworm infection is caused by a small, thin, white roundworm called Enterobius vermicularis. Although pinworom infection can affect all people, it most commonly occurs among children, institutionalized persons, and household members of persons with pinworm infection. Pinworm infection is treatable with over-the-counter or prescription medication, but reinfection, which occurs easily, should be prevented.

E. vermicularis

Image: Left: Adult male of E. vermicularis from a formalin-ethyl acetate (FEA) concentrated stool smear. The worm measured 1.4 mm in length. Image courtesy of Centre for Tropical Medicine and Imported Infectious Diseases. Right: Image of the eggs of the human parasite Enterobius vermicularis, or "human pinworm, " captured on cellulose tape under significant magnification. Credit: DPDx, PHIL.

Fascioliasis

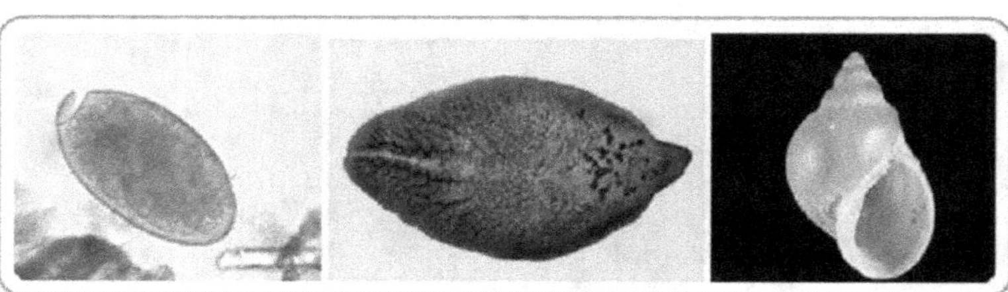

Fascioliasis is a parasitic infection typically caused by Fasciola hepatica, which is also known as "the common liver fluke" or "the sheep liver fluke." A related parasite, Fasciola gigantica, also can infect people. Fascioliasis is found in all continents except Antarctica, in over 70 countries, especially where there are sheep or cattle. People usually become infected by eating raw watercress or other water plants contaminated with immature parasite larvae. The young worms move through the intestinal wall, the abdominal cavity, and the liver tissue, into the bile ducts, where they develop into mature adult flukes that produce eggs. The pathology typically is most pronounced in the bile ducts and liver. Fasciola infection is both treatable and preventable.

Above Images: Left: Fasciola hepatica egg in an unstained wet mount (400x magnification). F. hepatica eggs are broadly ellipsoidal, operculated, and measure 130–150 μm by 60–90 μm. Center: Adult Fasciola hepatica fluke stained with carmine (30mm x 13mm). Right: Fossaria bulamoides, a snail host for F. hepatica in the western United States. (Credit: DPDx; Conchology, Inc., Mactan Island, Philippines)

Fasciolopsis buski

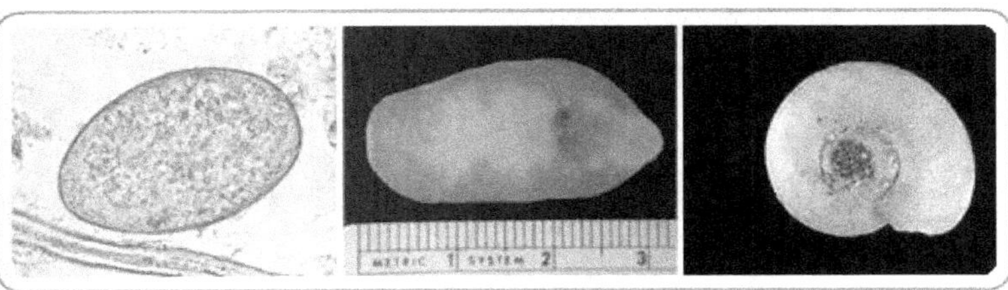

The intestinal fluke Fasciolopsis buski, which causes faciolopsiasis, is the largest intestinal fluke of humans. Fasciolopsiasis can be prevented by cooking aquatic plants well before eating them. Fasciolopsis is found in south and southeastern Asia. Fasciolopsiasis is treatable.

Image: Left: Fasciolopsis buski egg in an unstained wet mount. Center: Adult fluke of F. buski next to a scale. Right: Snail in the genus Hippeutis, an intermediate host for F. buski. Credit: DPDx, Image courtesy of Conchology, Inc, Mactan Island, Philippines.

Lymphatic Filariasis

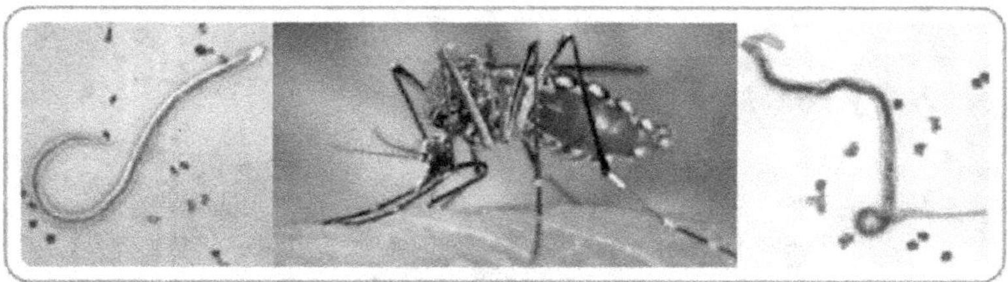

Lymphatic filariasis, considered globally as a neglected tropical disease (NTD), is a parasitic disease caused by microscopic, thread-like worms. The adult worms only live in the human lymph system. The lymph system maintains the body's fluid balance and fights infections. Lymphatic filariasis is spread from person to person by mosquitoes.

People with the disease can suffer from lymphedema and elephantiasis and in men, swelling of the scrotum, called hydrocele. Lymphatic filariasis is a leading cause of permanent disability worldwide. Communities frequently shun and reject women and men disfigured by the disease. Affected people frequently are unable to work because of their disability, and this harms their families and their communities.

Image: Left: Microfilaria of Wuchereria bancrofti in thick blood smear stained with Giemsa. Right: Microfilaria of Brugia malayi in a thick blood smear, stained with Giemsa. Center: Photograph of a female Aedes aegypti mosquito as she was in the process of obtaining a "blood meal." Laboratory strains of Aedes aegypti can be infected with Brugia. Credit: DPDx, PHIL

Giardia

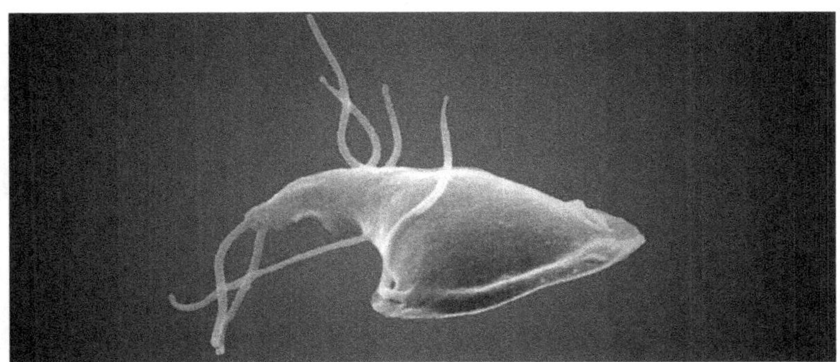

Giardia is a microscopic parasite that causes the diarrheal illness known as giardiasis. Giardia (also known as Giardia intestinalis, Giardia lamblia, or Giardia duodenalis) is found on surfaces or in soil, food, or water that has been contaminated with feces (poop) from infected humans or animals.

Giardia is protected by an outer shell that allows it to survive outside the body for long periods of time and makes it tolerant to chlorine disinfection. While the parasite can be spread in different ways, water (drinking water and recreational water) is the most common mode of transmission.

Gnathostomiasis (Gnathostoma Infection)

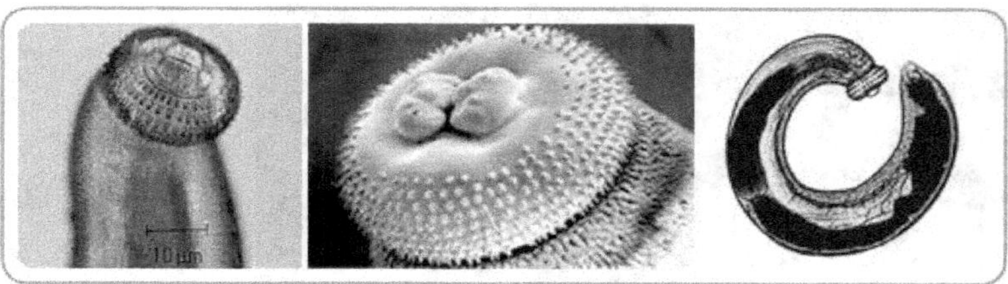

Human gnathostomiasis is caused by several species of parasitic worms (nematodes) in the genus Gnathostoma. The disease is found and is most commonly diagnosed in Southeast Asia, though it has also been found elsewhere in Asia, in South and Central America, and in some areas of Africa. People become infected primarily by eating undercooked or raw freshwater fish, eels, frogs, birds, and reptiles. The most common manifestations of the infection in humans are migratory swellings under the skin and increased levels of eosinophils in the blood. Rarely, the parasite can enter other tissues such as the liver, and the eye, resulting in vision loss or blindness, and the nerves, spinal cord, or brain, resulting in nerve pain, paralysis, coma and death.

Image: Left/Right: Third-stage larva of Gnathostoma spinigerum, head and whole larva respectively. Center: Scanning electron micrograph of a Gnathostoma spinigerum female worm's head bulb. Credit: DPDx

Adult head lice

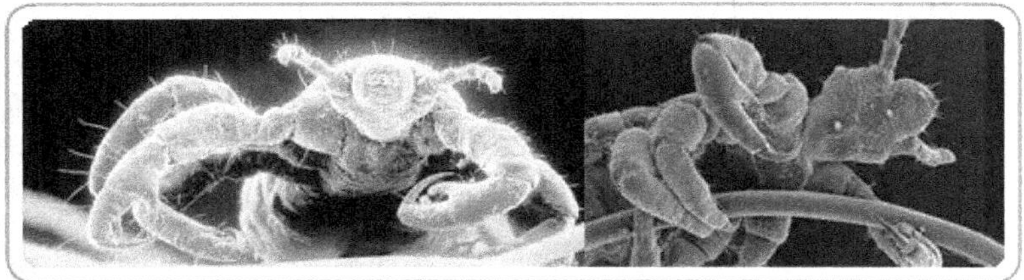

Adult head lice are roughly 2–3 mm long. Head lice infest the head and neck and attach their eggs to the base of the hair shaft. Lice move by crawling; they cannot hop or fly.
Head lice infestation, or pediculosis, is spread most commonly by close person-to-person contact. Dogs, cats, and other pets do not play a role in the transmission of human lice.

Both over-the-counter and prescription medications are available for treatment of head lice infestations.

Image: Two lice viewed under an electron microscope. Note the claws used to grasp onto individual hairs. Credit: CDC

Heterophyiasis
[Heterophyes heterophyes]

Causal Agents

The trematode Heterophyes heterophyes, a minute intestinal fluke.

Life Cycle

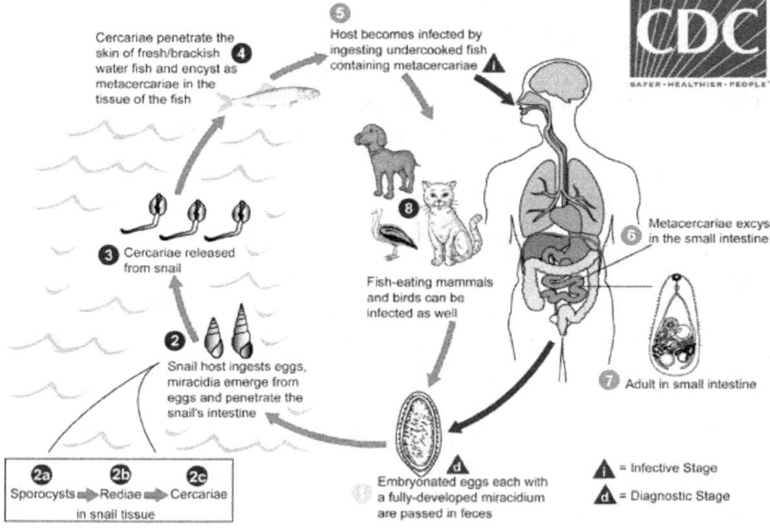

Hookworm

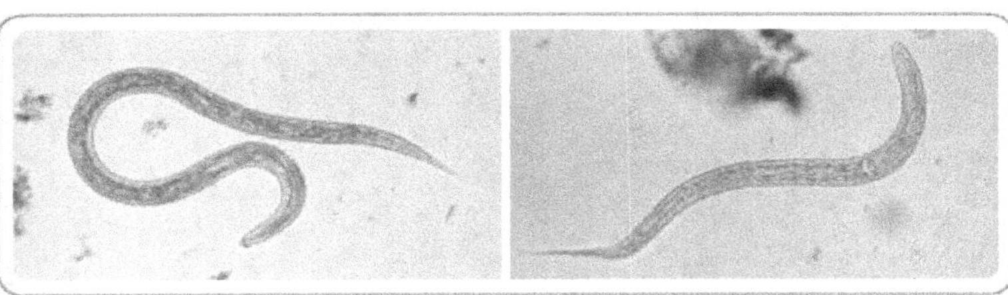

An estimated 576-740 million people in the world are infected with hookworm. Hookworm was once widespread in the United States, particularly in the southeastern region, but improvements in living conditions have greatly reduced hookworm infections. Hookworm, Ascaris, and whipworm are known as soil-transmitted helminths (parasitic worms). Together, they account for a major burden of disease worldwide.

Hookworms live in the small intestine. Hookworm eggs are passed in the feces of an infected person. If the infected person defecates outside (near bushes, in a garden, or field) of if the feces of an infected person are used as fertilizer, eggs are deposited on soil. They can then mature and hatch, releasing larvae (immature worms). The larvae mature into a form that can penetrate the skin of humans. Hookworm infection is mainly acquired by walking barefoot on contaminated soil. One kind of hookworm can also be transmitted through the ingestion of larvae.

Most people infected with hookworms have no symptoms. Some have gastrointestinal symptoms, especially persons who are infected for the first time. The most serious effects of hookworm infection are blood loss leading to anemia, in addition to protein loss. Hookworm infections are treatable with medication prescribed by your health care provider.

Image: L: Filariform (L3) hookworm larva in a wet mount. R: Hookworm rhabditiform larva (wet preparation). Credit: DPDx

Leishmaniasis

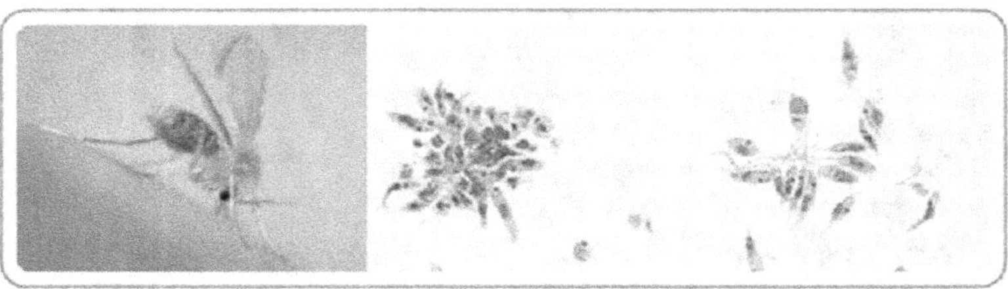

Leishmaniasis is a parasitic disease that is found in parts of the tropics, subtropics, and southern Europe. It is classified as a neglected tropical disease (NTD). Leishmaniasis is caused by infection with Leishmania parasites, which are spread by the bite of phlebotomine sand flies. There are several different forms of leishmaniasis in people. The most common forms are cutaneous leishmaniasis, which causes skin sores, and visceral leishmaniasis, which affects several internal organs (usually spleen, liver, and bone marrow).

Image: On average, the sand flies that transmit Leishmania are only about one-fourth the size of mosquitoes or even smaller. Left: Example of a vector sand fly (Phlebotomus papatasi) with a visible blood meal. Right: Leishmania promastigotes from a culture. The flagellated promastigote stage of the parasite is found in sand flies and in cultures. Credit: PHIL, DPDx

Liver Flukes

Liver flukes are parasites that can infect humans and cause liver and bile duct disease. There are two families of liver flukes that cause disease in humans: Opisthorchiidae (which includes species of Clonorchis and Opisthorchis) and Fasciolidae (which includes species of Fasciola). These two families of liver flukes differ in their geographic distribution, life cycle, and long-term outcome after clinical infection.

Loiasis

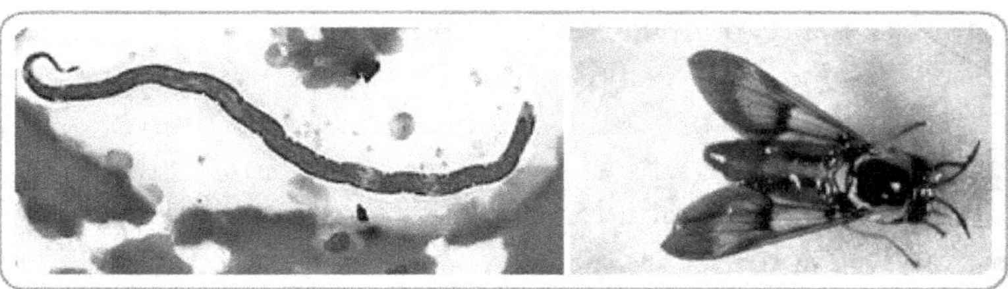

Loiasis, called African eye worm by most people, is caused by the parasitic worm Loa loa. It is passed on to humans through the repeated bites of deerflies (also known as mango flies or mangrove flies) of the genus Chrysops. The flies that pass on the parasite breed in certain rain forests of West and Central Africa. Infection with the parasite can also cause repeated episodes of itchy swellings of the body known as Calabar swellings. Knowing whether someone has a Loa loa infection has become more important in Africa because the presence of people with Loa loa infection has limited programs to control or eliminate onchocerciasis (river blindness) and lymphatic filariasis (elephantiasis). There may be more than 29 million people who are at risk of getting loaisis in affected areas of Central and West Africa.

Image: L: Microfilaria of L. loa in a thin blood smear, stained with Giemsa. R: Picture of Chrysops silacea feeding on a volunteer. Credit: DPDx

Lymphatic Filariasis

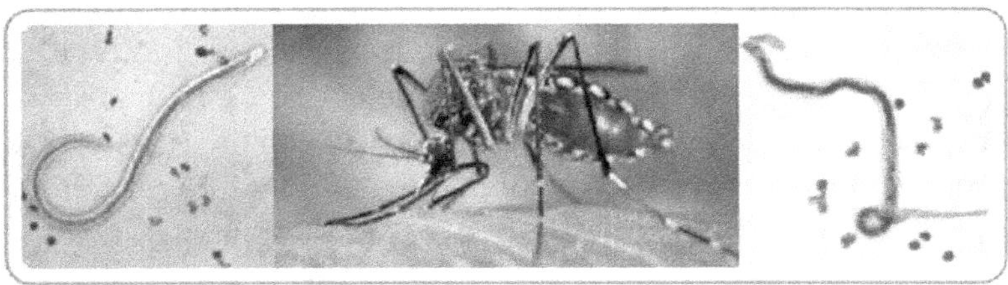

Lymphatic filariasis, considered globally as a neglected tropical disease (NTD), is a parasitic disease caused by microscopic, thread-like worms. The adult worms only live in the human lymph system. The lymph system maintains the body's fluid balance and fights infections. Lymphatic filariasis is spread from person to person by mosquitoes.
People with the disease can suffer from lymphedema and elephantiasis and in men, swelling of the scrotum, called hydrocele. Lymphatic filariasis is a leading cause of permanent disability worldwide. Communities frequently shun and reject women and men disfigured by the disease. Affected people frequently are unable to work because of their disability, and this harms their families and their communities.

Image: Left: Microfilaria of Wuchereria bancrofti in thick blood smear stained with Giemsa. Right: Microfilaria of Brugia malayi in a thick blood smear, stained with Giemsa. Center: Photograph of a female Aedes aegypti mosquito as she was in the process of obtaining a "blood meal." Laboratory strains of Aedes aegypti can be infected with Brugia. Credit: DPDx, PHIL

Malaria is a mosquito-borne disease caused by a parasite. People with malaria often experience fever, chills, and flu-like illness. Left untreated, they may develop severe complications and die. In 2017 an estimated 219 million cases of malaria occurred worldwide and 435,000 people died, mostly children in the African Region. About 1,700 cases of malaria are diagnosed in the United States each year. Many cases in the United States are in travelers and immigrants returning from countries where malaria transmission occurs, many from sub-Saharan Africa and South Asia.

Microsporidiosis

Causal Agents

The microsporidia are a group of unicellular intracellular parasites closely related to fungi, although the nature of the relation to the kingdom Fungi is not clear. The taxonomic position of this group has been debated and revised repeatedly; historically, they were considered protozoa and often remain managed by diagnostic parasitology laboratories. Microsporidia are characterized by the production of resistant spores that vary in size (usually 1—4 μm for medically-important species). They possess a unique organelle, the polar tubule or polar filament, which is coiled inside the spore as demonstrated by its ultrastructure. Microsporidia also possess degenerated mitochondria called mitosomes and lack a conventional Golgi apparatus.

Human scabies

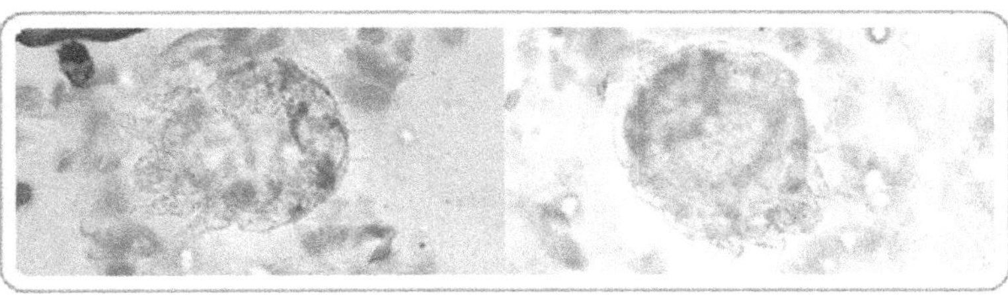

Human scabies is caused by an infestation of the skin by the human itch mite (Sarcoptes scabiei var. hominis). The microscopic scabies mite burrows into the upper layer of the skin where it lives and lays its eggs. The most common symptoms of scabies are intense itching and a pimple-like skin rash. The scabies mite usually is spread by direct, prolonged; skin-to-skin contact with a person who has scabies.

Scabies occurs worldwide and affects people of all races and social classes. Scabies can spread rapidly under crowded conditions where close body contact is frequent. Institutions such as nursing homes, extended-care facilities, and prisons are often sites of scabies outbreaks.

Image: Sarcoptes scabiei mites in a skin scraping, stained with lactophenol cotton-blue. Credit: DPDx

Myiasis

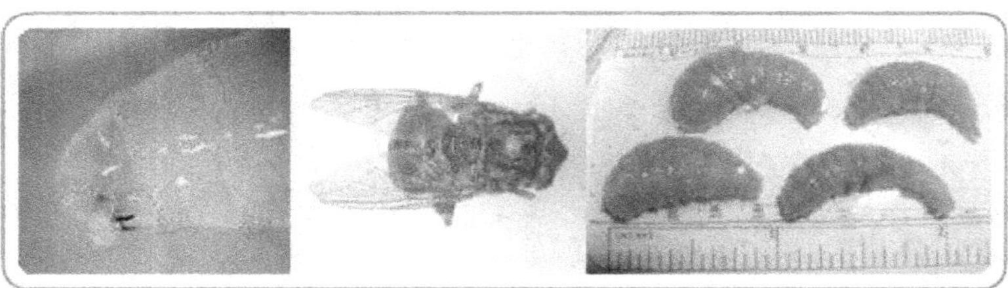

Myiasis is the infection of a fly larva (maggot) in human tissue. This occurs in tropical and subtropical areas. Myiasis is rarely acquired in the United States; people typically get the infection when they travel to tropical areas in Africa and South America. People traveling with untreated and open wounds are more at risk for getting myiasis. Fly larvae need to be surgically removed by a medical professional.

Image: L to R: Close-up of the anterior end of a larva, showing the mandibles and one of the anterior spiracles. Adult of Dermatobia hominis, the human bot fly. Four larvae of Dermatobia hominis, removed from a human host. DPDx, Georgia Museum of Natural History.

Naegleria fowleri

— Primary Amebic Meningoencephalitis (PAM) — Amebic Encephalitis

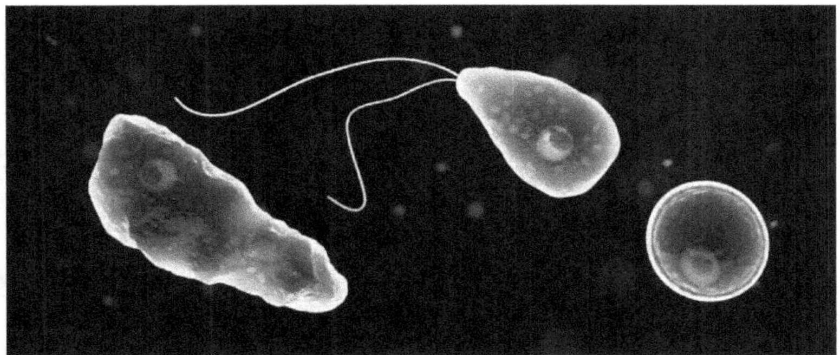

Naegleria fowleri (commonly referred to as the "brain-eating amoeba" or "brain-eating ameba"), is a free-living microscopic ameba*, (single-celled living organism). It can cause a rare** and devastating infection of the brain called primary amebic meningoencephalitis (PAM). The ameba is commonly found in warm freshwater (e.g. lakes, rivers, and hot springs) and soil. Naegleria fowleri usually infects people when contaminated water enters the body through the nose. Once the ameba enters the nose, it travels to the brain where it causes PAM, which is usually fatal. Infection typically occurs when people go swimming or diving in warm freshwater places, like lakes and rivers. In very rare instances, Naegleria infections may also occur when contaminated water from other sources (such as inadequately chlorinated swimming pool water or heated and contaminated tap water) enters the nose 1-4. You cannot get infected from swallowing water contaminated with Naegleria.

Top image (from left to right): Computer-generated representation of Naegleria fowleri in its ameboid trophozoite stage, in its flagellated stage, and in its cyst stage.

Toxocariasis (also known as Roundworm Infection)

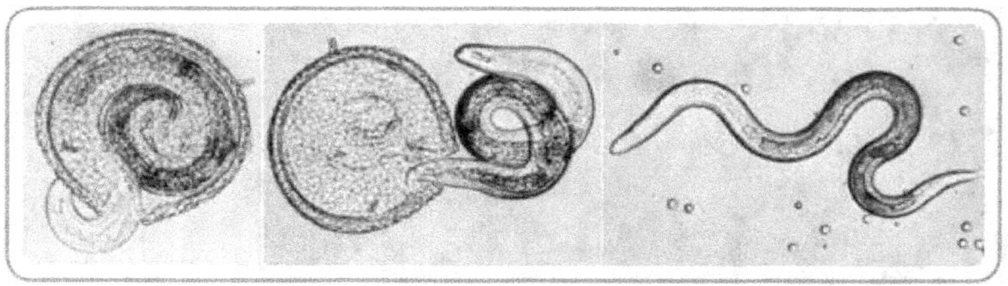

Toxocariasis is the parasitic disease caused by the larvae of two species of Toxocara roundworms: Toxocara canis from dogs and, less commonly, Toxocara cati from cats. Toxocariasis is considered one of the Neglected Parasitic Infections, a group of five parasitic diseases that have been targeted by CDC for public health action.

Image: Various stages of Toxocara canis larva hatching. Credit: DPDx

Onchocerciasis (also known as River Blindness)

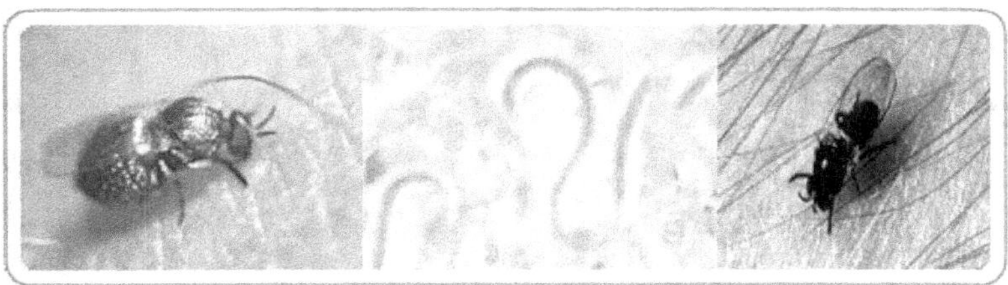

Onchocerciasis, or River Blindness, is a neglected tropical disease (NTD) caused by the parasitic worm Onchocerca volvulus. It is transmitted through repeated bites by blackflies of the genus Simulium. The disease is called River Blindness because the blackfly that transmits the infection lives and breeds near fast-flowing streams and rivers and the infection can result in blindness. In addition to visual impairment or blindness, onchocerciasis causes skin disease, including nodules under the skin or debilitating itching. Worldwide onchocerciasis is second only to trachoma as an infectious cause of blindness.

Image: Left/Right: Blackflies, the vector of onchocerciasis. Center: Microfilariae of O. volvulus from a skin nodule of a patient from Zambia, stained with H&E. Image taken at 1000x oil magnification. Credit: WHOExternal, DPDx, CDC

Opisthorchis Infection

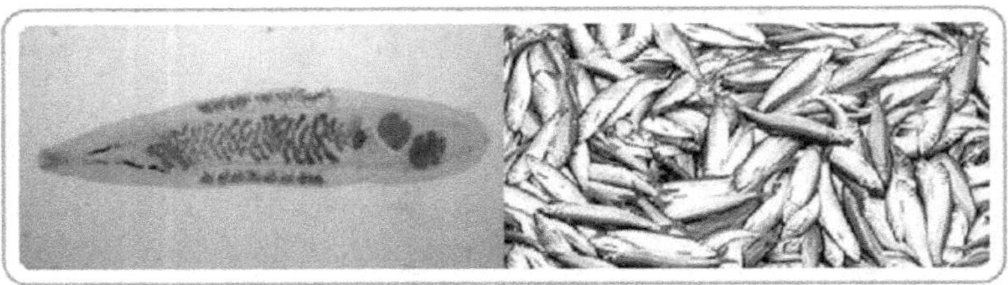

Opisthorchis species are liver fluke parasites that humans can get by eating raw or undercooked fish, crabs, or crayfish from areas in Asia and Europe where the parasite is found, including Thailand, Laos, Cambodia, Vietnam, Germany, Italy, Belarus, Russia, Kazakhstan, and Ukraine. Liver flukes infect the liver, gallbladder, and bile duct in humans. While most infected persons do not show any symptoms, infections that last a long time can result in severe symptoms and serious illness. Untreated, infections may persist for up to 25–30 years, the lifespan of the parasite. Typical symptoms include indigestion, abdominal pain, diarrhea, or constipation. In severe cases, abdominal pain, nausea, and diarrhea can occur. O. felineus, in addition to presenting with the typical symptoms also seen in O. viverrini infections, can present with fever, facial swelling, swollen lymph glands, sore joints, and rash—similar to the signs and symptoms of schistosomiasis. Chronic O. felineus infections may also involve the pancreatic ducts.Diagnosis of Opisthorchis infection is based on microscopic identification of parasite eggs in stool specimens. Safe and effective medication is available to treat Opisthorchis infections. Adequately freezing or cooking fish will kill the parasite.

Above Images: Left: Adult of O. felineus. Right: A large group of fish. Fish do not have to ingest anything to become infected because the parasite can infect fish under the scales or through the flesh. Eating infected fish can result in Opisthorchis infection. (Credit: Web Atlas of Medical Parasitology and the Korean Society for Parasitology, NEFSC/NOAAExternal)

Paragonimus

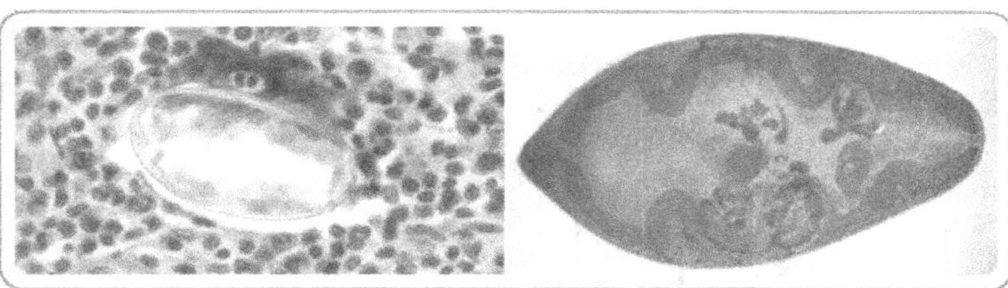

Paragonimus is a lung fluke (flatworm) that infects the lungs of humans after eating an infected raw or undercooked crab or crayfish. Less frequent, but more serious cases of paragonimiasis occur when the parasite travels to the central nervous system.

Although rare, paragonimiasis has been acquired in the United States, with multiple cases reported from the Midwest. Once the diagnosis is made, effective treatment for paragonimiasis is available from a physician.

Image: Left: Eggs of Paragonimus sp. taken from a lung biopsy stained with hematoxylin and eosin (H&E). These eggs measured 80-90 μm by 40-45 μm. The species was not identified in this case. Right: P. westermani adult, this approximately 1cm long fluke is viewed under magnification. Credit: DPDx

Sarcocystosis

Sarcocystosis is a disease caused by a microscopic parasite Sarcocystis. In humans, two types of the disease can occur, one causes diarrhea, mild fever, and vomiting (intestinal type), and the other type causes muscle pain, transitory edema, and fever (muscular type). However, most people infected with Sarcocystis do not have symptoms. Sarcocystosis occurs in tropical or subtropical countries. Muscular sarcocystosis has most often been reported from countries in Southeast Asia.

Sporulated oocysts of Sarcocystis sp. in a wet mount viewed under UV microscopy, magnification 400x. Credit: DPDx

Soil-transmitted helminths

Soil-transmitted helminths refer to the intestinal worms infecting humans that are transmitted through contaminated soil ("helminth" means parasitic worm): Ascaris lumbricoides (sometimes called just "Ascaris"), whipworm (Trichuris trichiura), and hookworm (Anclostoma duodenale and Necator americanus). A large part of the world's population is infected with one or more of these soil-transmitted helminths:

approximately 807-1,121 million with Ascaris
approximately 604-795 million with whipworm
approximately 576-740 million with hookworm
Soil-transmitted helminth infection is found mainly in areas with warm and moist climates where sanitation and hygiene are poor, including in temperate zones during warmer months. These STHs are considered Neglected Tropical Diseases (NTDs) because they inflict tremendous disability and suffering yet can be controlled or eliminated.

Soil-transmitted helminths live in the intestine and their eggs are passed in the feces of infected persons. If an infected person defecates outside (near bushes, in a garden, or field) or if the feces of an infected person are used as fertilizer, eggs are deposited on soil. Ascaris and hookworm eggs become infective as they mature in soil. People are infected with Ascaris and whipworm when eggs are ingested. This can happen when hands or fingers that have contaminated dirt on them are put in the mouth or by consuming vegetables and fruits that have not been carefully cooked, washed or peeled. Hookworm eggs are not infective. They hatch in soil, releasing larvae (immature worms) that mature into a form that can penetrate the skin of humans. Hookworm infection is transmitted primarily by walking barefoot on contaminated soil. One kind of hookworm (Anclostoma duodenale) can also be transmitted through the ingestion of larvae.

People with light soil-transmitted helminth infections usually have no symptoms. Heavy infections can cause a range of health problems, including abdominal pain, diarrhea, blood and protein loss, rectal prolapse, and physical and cognitive growth retardation. Soil-transmitted helminth infections are treatable with medication prescribed by your health care provider.

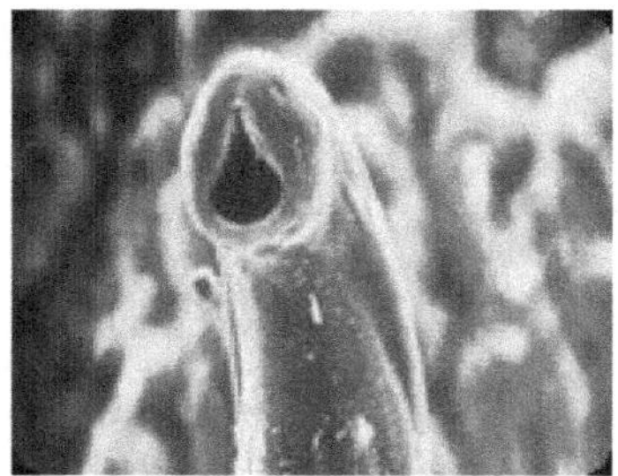

An estimated 576-740 million people in the world are infected with hookworm. Hookworm was widespread in the southeastern United States until the early 20th century but is now nearly eliminated. Hookworm, Ascaris, and whipworm are known as soil-transmitted helminths (parasitic worms). Together, they account for a major burden of disease worldwide.

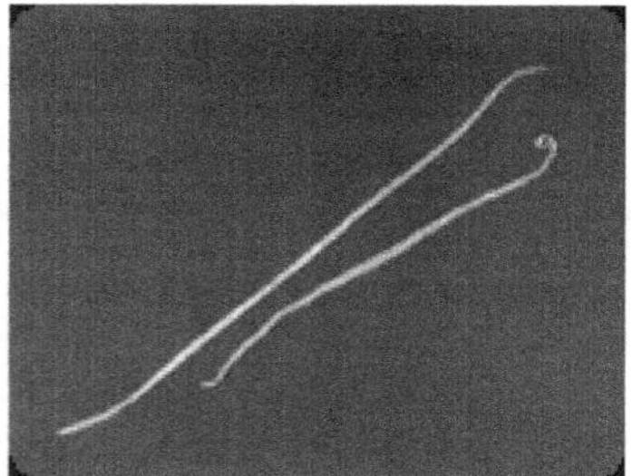

An estimated 807-1,221 million people in the world are infected with Ascaris lumbricoides (sometimes called just "Ascaris"). Ascaris, hookworm, and whipworm are known as soil-transmitted helminths (parasitic worms). Together, they account for a major burden of disease worldwide. Ascariasis is now uncommon in the United States.

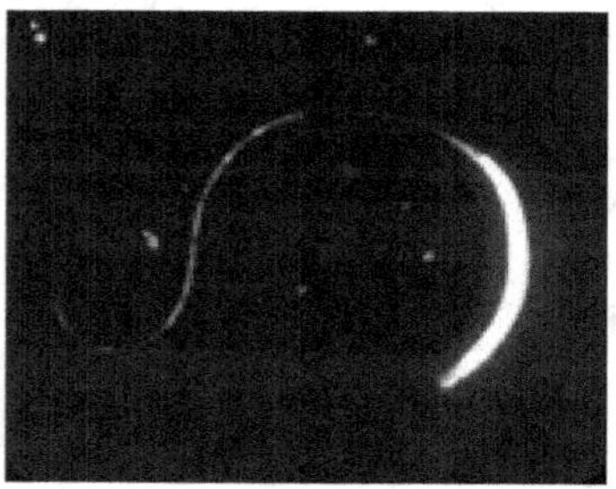

An estimated 604-795 million people in the world are infected with whipworm. Whipworm, hookworm, and Ascaris are known as soil-transmitted helminths (parasitic worms). Together, they account for a major burden of disease worldwide.

Strongyloides

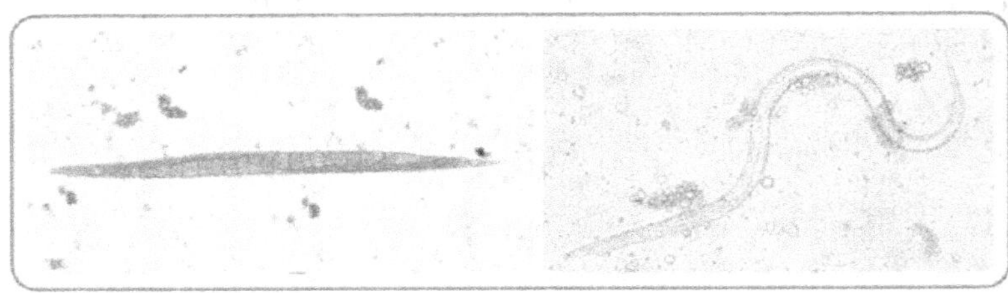

Strongyloidiasis was first described in French troops who had returned from modern day Vietnam during the late 19th century who were suffering from severe, persistent diarrhea. It is a parasitic disease caused by nematodes, or roundworms, in the genus Strongyloides. The parasites enter the body through exposed skin, such as bare feet. Strongyloides is most common in tropical or subtropical climates.

Most people who are infected with Strongyloides do not know they are infected and have no symptoms. Others, particularly those who are on some immunosuppressive therapies, may develop a severe form and, if untreated, become critically ill and possibly die.

Above Images: Left: Adult free-living female S. stercoralis. Notice the row of eggs within the female's body. Right: Filariform (L3) larva of S. stercoralis in an unstained wet mount. Credit: DPDx.

Taeniasis

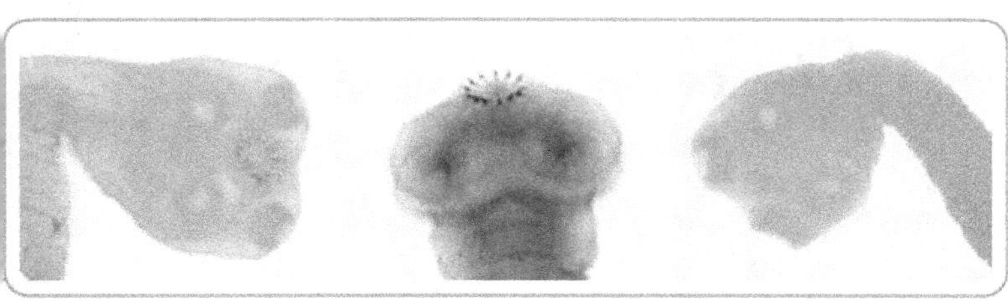

Taeniasis in humans is a parasitic infection caused by the tapeworm species Taenia saginata (beef tapeworm), Taenia solium (pork tapeworm), and Taenia asiatica (Asian tapeworm). Humans can become infected with these tapeworms by eating raw or undercooked beef (T. saginata) or pork (T. solium and T. asiatica). People with taeniasis may not know they have a tapeworm infection because symptoms are usually mild or nonexistent. Taenia solium tapeworm infections can lead to cysticercosis, which is a disease that can cause seizures, so it is important seek treatment.

Image: L&C: Scoleces of T. solium. Note the four large suckers and rostellum containing two rows of hooks. R: Scolex of T. saginata. Note the four large suckers and lack of rostellum and rostellar hooks. Credit: DPDx

Toxoplasmosis (Toxoplasma infection)

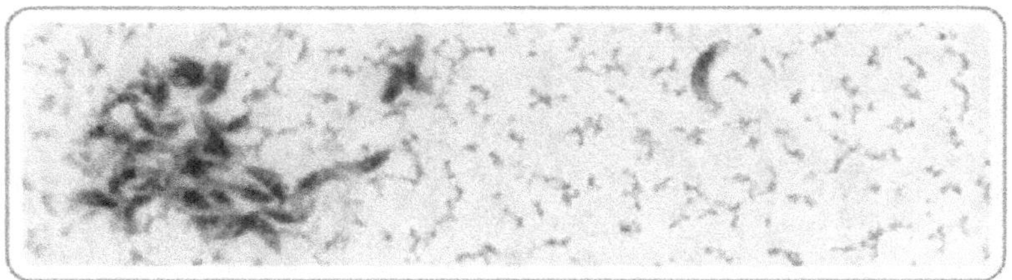

Toxoplasmosis is considered to be a leading cause of death attributed to foodborne illness in the United States. More than 40 million men, women, and children in the U.S. carry the Toxoplasma parasite, but very few have symptoms because the immune system usually keeps the parasite from causing illness.However, women newly infected with Toxoplasma during or shortly before pregnancy and anyone with a compromised immune system should be aware that toxoplasmosis can have severe consequences. Toxoplasmosis is considered one of the neglected parasitic infections of the United States, a group of five parasitic diseases that have been targeted by CDC for public health action. Image: Toxoplasma gondii in mouse ascitic fluid. Smear. (Credit: DPDx)

Trichinellosis (also known as Trichinosis)

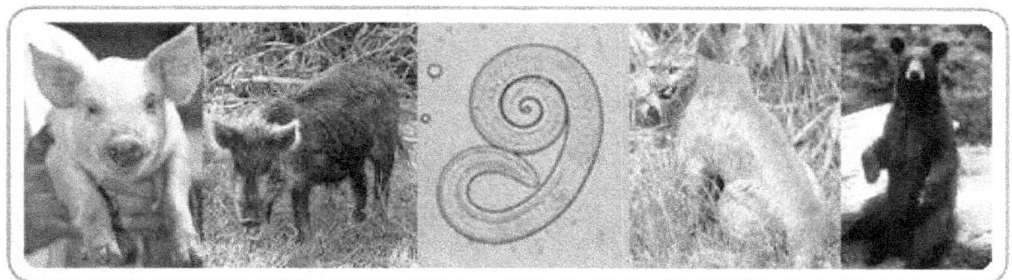

Trichinellosis, also called trichinosis, is a disease that people can get by eating raw or undercooked meat from animals infected with the microscopic parasite Trichinella.

Image: Center: Trichinella larva in muscle tissue from an Alaskan bear. Image photographed at 200x magnification. L/R: Pigs, feral hogs, cougars and black bears can all harbor Trichinella infection. Successful trichinae control programs by the U.S. pork industry have nearly eliminated the disease in domestic swine raised in confinement, but hogs raised outdoors in close contact with rodents and other wildlife have an increased chance of acquiring Trichinella infection.

Credit: L to R: USDAExternal, NASA/KSCExternal, DPDx, U.S. Fish & Wildlife ServiceExternal

Trichuriasis (also known as Whipworm Infection)

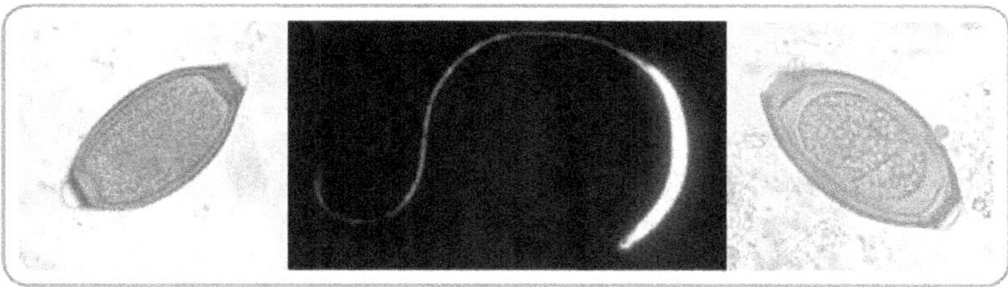

An estimated 604-795 million people in the world are infected with whipworm. Whipworm, hookworm, and Ascaris are known as soil-transmitted helminths (parasitic worms). Together, they account for a major burden of disease worldwide.

Whipworms live in the large intestine and whipworm eggs are passed in the feces of infected persons. If the infected person defecates outside (near bushes, in a garden, or field) or if human feces as used as fertilizer, eggs are deposited on soil. They can then mature into a form that is infective. Whipworm infection is caused by ingesting eggs. This can happen when hands or fingers that have contaminated dirt on them are put in the mouth or by consuming vegetables or fruits that have not been carefully cooked, washed or peeled.

People infected with whipworm can suffer light or heavy infections. People with light infections usually have no symptoms. People with heavy symptoms can experience frequent, painful passage of stool that contains a mixture of mucus, water, and blood. Rectal prolapse can also occur. Children with heavy infections can become severely anemic and growth-retarded. Whipworm infections are treatable with medication prescribed by your health care provider.

Image: Left: Egg of T. trichiura in an iodine-stained wet mount. Right: Egg of T. trichiura in an unstained wet mount. Center: Micrograph of an adult female Trichuris human whipworm that is approximately 4cm long. Credit: DPDx, PHIL.

www.ingramcontent.com/pod-product-compliance
Lightning Source LLC
Chambersburg PA
CBHW061351250726
48657CB00004B/1441